IRRITABLE BOWEL SYNDROME - NOVEL CONCEPTS FOR RESEARCH AND TREATMENT

Edited by **Victor Chaban**

Irritable Bowel Syndrome - Novel Concepts for Research and Treatment
http://dx.doi.org/10.5772/62930
Edited by Victor Chaban

Contributors

Mihaela Fadgyas Stanculete, Francesca Pasqui, Carolina Poli, Caterina Magrino, Davide Festi, Elsa Eriksson, Kristina Andrén, Henry Eriksson, Alexandra Chira, Romeo Ioan Chira, Dan Lucian Dumitrascu, Victor Chaban

Published by InTech

Janeza Trdine 9, 51000 Rijeka, Croatia

Publishing Process Manager Iva Simcic

Technical Editor SPi Global

Cover InTech Design team

First published January, 2017

Printed in Croatia

Additional hard copies can be obtained from orders@intechopen.com

Irritable Bowel Syndrome - Novel Concepts for Research and Treatment, Edited by Victor Chaban

p. cm.

Print ISBN 978-953-51-2827-4
Online ISBN 978-953-51-2828-1

For EU product safety concerns:
IN TECH d.o.o., Prolaz Marije Krucifikse Kozulić 3, 51000 Rijeka, Croatia, info@intechopen.com or visit our website at intechopen.com.

Meet the editor

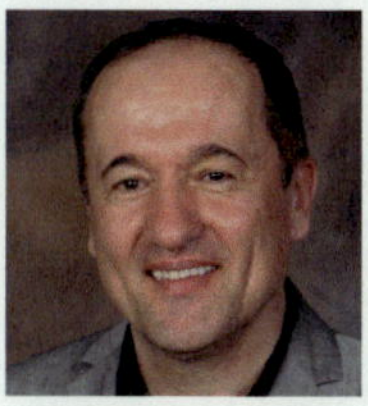

Dr. Victor V. Chaban is a professor of Medicine with dual faculty appointment at Charles R. Drew University (CDU) of Medicine and Science and the University of California, Los Angeles (UCLA). Dr. Chaban completed his postdoctoral training in Neuroscience at UCLA and graduate studies in Clinical Research at CDU. His area of expertise is signal transduction mechanisms of nociception associated with clinical presentations of visceral pain. Dr. Chaban is a member of the US National Institutes of Health and several international study sections. For his service and scientific work, Dr. Chaban received the President's Award for Excellence in Service to CDU. Currently, Dr. Chaban is an associate editor for *Anatomy and Applied Physiology*, executive editor for *Journal of Autacoids and Hormones*, and editor in chief for the *International Journal of Research in Nursing*.

Contents

Preface

Defining sites for new interventions for irritable bowel syndrome (IBS) will have a significant impact on society with possible successful translations of basic and clinical studies into new therapies. Over the last decade, medical literature has documented the undertreatment of IBS, which affects up to 25% of population worldwide. As a result, the new data presented in this book will meet public concerns and also will be an important resource for investigators performing clinical research studies, as well as healthcare providers and patients suffering from this disorder.

The hypothesis that the central nervous system and gastrointestinal system are closely connected is widely accepted, and we signified this concept in this book by presenting an overview of IBS as a functional gastrointestinal disorder regulated by the nervous system. In addition to enteric nervous system regulation, this disorder often is accompanied by changes in the central nervous system such as concomitant decline in cognitive or motor performance. In this book, we provide an overlook of psychotropic treatment to compare the efficacy of various available drugs. Pain that in some patients is out of proportion to identifiable pathology is the most common, immediate, and dramatic consequence of IBS and is responsible for a highly negative impact on quality of life. Primary afferent neurons, smooth muscles, and other cells of the affected tissues may interact in a cell-to-cell manner messages through the transfer of hormones, cytokines, and other mediators that influence normal functioning. The complex interplay and balance between these diverse mediators, aging, genetic background, and environmental factors may ultimately determine the outcome of progression of IBS.

IBS pathology is further illustrated by the fact that the average time duration between the onset of this disorder and the diagnosis can take many years. One of the key features for effective treatment is to look for comorbidity with other diseases in patient evaluations. In view of the iatrogenic component in the maintenance of functional somatic syndromes of IBS, doctor-centered interventions and close observation of the doctor-patient relationship are of particular importance. Those cases tending to trigger IBS include food content, food allergies or food intolerance, and the role of gut inflammation.

It is impossible to give an overview of all aspects of IBS; however, this book represents current research in the study of the symptoms, diagnosis, mechanisms, and treatment options for IBS. Topics discussed are valuable resource for clinicians, students, and scientists and are recommended for healthcare providers seeking new insights into therapies, as well as patients suffering from IBS.

Dr. Victor Chaban, Professor
Department of Internal Medicine, Charles R. Drew University of Medicine and Science
Department of Medicine, University of California
Los Angeles, USA

Chapter 1

Irritable Bowel Syndrome: Functional Gastrointestinal Disease Regulated by Nervous System

Victor V. Chaban

Additional information is available at the end of the chapter

http://dx.doi.org/10.5772/112443

Abstract

A functional disorder is a medical condition that impairs the normal function, but without major organic cause such as irritation or inflammation and where the organ or part of the body looks completely normal under medical examination. The accumulation of abnormalities that limit body functions is a major risk factor for patients with irritable bowel syndrome (IBS), defined as a gastrointestinal disorder with abdominal pain or discomfort that is associated with a change in bowel habit. Often, this disorder is accompanied by the concomitant decline in cognitive or motor performance. Pain that in some patients is out of proportion to identifiable pathology is the most immediate and dramatic consequence of IBS and is responsible for a highly negative impact on quality of life and substantial workforce loss. For patients with IBS, the most common comorbid diagnoses include painful bladder syndrome (PBS) or chronic pelvic pain (CPP). Cells of the affected tissues may interact in cell-to-cell manner messages through the transfer of hormones, cytokines, and other mediators that influence normal functioning. The complex interplay and balance between these diverse mediators, ageing, genetic background, and environmental factors may ultimately determine the outcome of the progression of the functional disorder. On a cellular level, these responses are highly complex, involving a vast array of enzymes and receptors of virtually every class, directing recruitment of many types of cells to recover the healthy state. Indeed, a balance between the messengers with the inherent redundancy of the different body systems makes therapeutic intervention of functional disorders a considerable challenge.

Keywords: sensory neurons, extrinsic primary afferents, nociception

1. Introduction

The response properties of pelvic extrinsic primary afferent nerves (EPANs) play an important role in etiology of irritable bowel syndrome (IBS). Hypersensitivity of visceral mechanoreceptors could result from excessive production of modulatory neurotransmitters. In addition to direct stimulation of stretch-activated channels on primary afferent neurons located in dorsal root ganglia (DRG), chemicals produced by different target cells (such as smooth muscle cells and interstitial cells of Cajal) in response to stretch or inflammation play an important role in the neuromodulation of nociception. The incidence of persistent, episodic, or chronic visceral pain is more prevalent in females, which also suggests hormonal regulation. Despite extensive research of the properties of pelvic and splanchnic afferent nerves, little is known about the mechanisms underlying normal and pathological signal transduction pathways underlying many functional diseases. Despite considerable efforts by the scientific community and the pharmaceutical industry to develop novel pharmacological treatments aimed at chronic visceral pain, the traditional approaches to identifying and evaluating novel drugs for this target have largely failed to translate into effective IBS treatments [1]. A better understanding of these processes has direct implications for the development of more effective therapies. During the last decade, we identified that DRG neurons can be affected by ATP, NO, estrogen, and other mediators producing neuronal hyper- or desensitization that may unravel the enigma of the development of chronic pelvic pain associated with IBS. Moreover, our recent data that estrogen can gate primary afferent response to modulate nociception support the idea about involvement of peripheral central system in etiology of a wide range of the functional and inflammatory gastrointestinal diseases [2].

2. Role of EPANs in the mechanisms of visceral neurotransduction and modulation

Pelvic nerve afferent fibers innervating the visceral organs of the lower colon have been well characterized (reviewed in Ref. [3]). In general, during colonic distension, a large number of pelvic EPANs show static levels of discharge. Stretches that lead to the opening of stretch-activated (SA) channels on the plasma membrane lead to the selective or nonselective opening of different cation and anion channels in nodose ganglia and DRG neurons. Thus, depending on the cell type and channel type, EPANs activation may result in hyperpolarization, depolarization, or primarily Ca^{2+} influx. The function of SA channels in the plasma membrane differs between various cell types. Influx of Ca^{2+} may repolarize the plasma membrane via activation of K_{ca} channels and inactivating of voltage-gated calcium channels (VGCCs), and thus influence adaptation rates of sensory neurons during ongoing stimulations.

The cell bodies of primary visceral spinal afferent neurons are located in the lumbosacral (L1-S1) DRGs that transmit information about chemical or mechanical stimulation from the periphery to the spinal cord. Nociceptors are small- to medium-size DRG neurons whose peripheral processes detect potentially damaging physical and chemical stimuli. Until recently, ATP release from nonneuronal cells was thought to be exclusively as result of injury. It is now clear that certain integral membrane proteins contain an ATP-binding cassette so this

http://dx.doi.org/10.5772/112443

neurotransmitter can act as signaling molecule modulating sensory afferent nerve terminals. Six P2X receptors are expressed in DRGs. Significantly, the P2X3 receptor is found exclusively in a subset of small diameter capsaicin sensitive peripheral sensory neurons (presumably nociceptors) [4]. Today, multiple lines of evidence suggest that ATP signaling via P2X receptors contribute to different pain phenotypes, therefore P2X antagonists may be useful analgesics. The availability of P2X receptor-specific antagonists also holds the promise of revealing the cellular and molecular neurobiology underlying pain states underlying functional diseases [5]. With sufficiently high levels of ATP, P2X and SA channels (which has a greater permeability for Ca^{2+} than Na^{+}) would depolarize nerve terminals directly producing action potentials and leading to sensation of pain. On the other hand, the response of EPANs may be tonically inhibited by NO produced by peripheral nerve terminals. The peripheral sensitization of nerve fibers is transient depending on the duration of stimuli and the presence of visceral (colonic) inflammation.

3. Estrogen receptors and visceral nociception associated with functional diseases

Changes in pain perception and variations of symptoms throughout the menstrual cycle, as well as sexual intercourse triggering symptoms in a significant portion of females diagnosed with irritable bowel syndrome (IBS), painful bladder syndrome (PBS), chronic pelvic pain (CPP), and other function syndromes, points to a connection with sex steroids. Several lines of evidence indicate that 17β-estradiol (E2) directly influence the functions of primary afferent neurons. Both subtypes of estrogen receptors (ERα and ERβ) are present in DRG neurons including the small-diameter putative nociceptors [4]. In vitro, ATP-sensitive DRG neurons respond to E2 [6, 7], which correlated well with the idea that visceral afferents are E2 sensitive: (i) visceral pain is affected by hormonal level in cycling females; (ii) there are sex differences in the prevalence of functional disorders involving the viscera; and (iii) putative visceral afferents fit into the population of DRG neurons that are sensitive to E2 [7]. These data suggest that in addition to the CNS actions, E2 can act in the periphery to modulate nociception [6, 7]. E2 modulates cellular activity by altering ion channel opening, G-protein signaling, and activation of trophic factor-like signal transduction pathways. These effects have been ascribed to membrane-associated receptors [8]. The results from our laboratory and others indicate that E2 acts in DRG neurons to modulate L-type VGCC and through group II metabotropic glutamate receptors [6].

E2 has a significant role in modulating visceral sensitivity, indicating that E2 alterations in sensory processing may underlie sex-based differences in functional pain symptoms [9]. Indeed in most clinical studies, women report more severe pain levels, more frequent pain, and longer duration of pain than men [10]. Little is known about E2-mediated mechanisms in peripheral nervous system, but the fact that DRG neurons express ERs and respond to E2 treatment suggest that they are a potential target for mediating nociception. E2 modulation of nociceptive response depends on the type of pain, its durations, and the involvement of other nociceptive-mediated mechanisms.

E2 (both short-term and long-term exposure) significantly decreased the nociceptive signaling in viscerally labeled DRG neurons [6, 7]. Thus, in addition to central regulation, estrogen may affect nociception associated with IBS peripherally.

4. Primary afferent neurons and viscero-visceral cross-sensitization: emerging model for functional gastrointestinal disorders

Most of the current literature pertains to specific functional syndromes defined by medical subspecialties. These include: IBS (gastroenterology); CPP (gynecology); PBS (urology); fibromyalgia (rheumatology); and others. Many reports described the substantial overlaps between two or more of these syndromes [11, 12]. Moreover, clinical presentations of functional syndromes lack a specific pathology in the affected organ but may respond to a viscero-visceral cross-sensitization in which increased nociceptive input from an inflamed organ (i.e., uterus) sensitizes neurons that receive convergent input from an unaffected organ (i.e., colon or bladder). The site of visceral cross-sensitivity is unknown.

Recent studies from our laboratory demonstrated that hormonal modulation of visceral inputs of primary afferent nociceptors located in the dorsal root ganglia (DRG) is responsible for changes observed in the perception of pain during the etiology of functional pain syndromes [2]. Individuals suffering from CPP frequently have pain emanating from several visceral organs. Viscero-somatic and viscero-visceral hyperalgesia and allodynia lead to the perception of pain spreading from an initial site to adjacent areas. Patients with CPP may at first have only one source of pain in the pelvis, but numerous mechanisms involving the central and peripheral nervous systems may result in the development of painful sensations in adjacent organs, such as IBS being associated with lower colonic pain.

5. Summary

Similar to other chronic diseases, a multicomponent conceptual model of IBS, which involves physiologic, cognitive and behavior factors will be necessary for developing new therapies. The different systems such as neuroendocrine regulation, pain modulation, and autonomic response will affect ascending aminergic systems (**Figure 1**).

From a public health perspective, a substantial impact on our knowledge of nociceptive diseases such IBS will help achieve a deeper understanding of data presented in clinical aspects of these symptoms. Only a thorough understanding of the mechanism implicated in these phenomena can truly contribute to the designing of new and more efficient therapies.

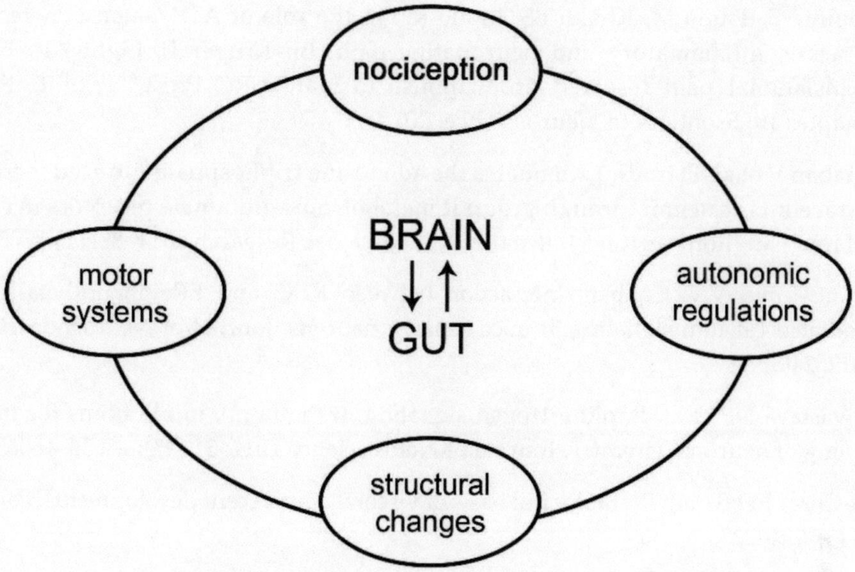

Figure 1. Different regulatory mechanisms involved in irritable bowel syndrome.

Author details

Victor V. Chaban

Address all correspondence to: victorchaban@cdrewu.edu

Department of Internal Medicine, Charles R. Drew University of Medicine and Science, Los Angeles, USA; Department of Medicine, University of California, Los Angeles, USA

References

[1] Holschneider DP, Bradesi S, Mayer EA. The role of experimental models in developing new treatments for irritable bowel syndrome. Expert Review of Gastroenterology and Hepatology, 2011, 5 (1): 43–57.

[2] Chaban V. Unraveling the enigma of visceral pain. Nova Publishers, N.Y. 2016. 77 p. ISBN: 978-63489-430-8. Library of U.S. Congress Control Number: 2015951299.

[3] Mayer EA, Labus JS, Tillisch K, Cole SW, Baldi P Towards a systems view of IBS. Nature Review Gastroenterology and Hepatology 2015, 12 (10): 592–605.

[4] Kobayashi K, Yamanaka H, Noguchi K. Expression of ATP receptors in the rat dorsal root ganglion and spinal cord. Anatomical Science International 2013, 88 (1): 10–16.

[5] Toulme E, Tsuda M, Khakh BS, Inoue K. On the role of ATP-Gated P2X receptors in acute, inflammatory and neuropathic pain. In: Kruger L, Light AR, Editors. Translational pain research: from mouse to man. CRC Press/Taylor & Francis. Chapter 10. Frontiers in Neuroscience. 2010.

[6] Chaban V et al. Estradiol attenuates the adenosine triphosphate-induced increase of intracellular calcium through group II metabotropic glutamate receptors in rat dorsal root ganglion neurons. Journal of Neuroscience Research 2011. 89(11):1707–1710.

[7] Cho, T. and V.V. Chaban, Interaction between P2X3 and ERalpha/ERbeta in ATP-mediated calcium signaling in mice sensory neurons. Journal of Neuroendocrinology 2012. 24(5): 789–97

[8] Srivastava DP et al. Rapid estrogen signaling in the brain: implications for the fine-tuning of neuronal circuitry. Journal of Neuroscience 2011. 31 (45): 16056–16063.

[9] Al-Chaer ED, Traub RJ. Biological basis of visceral pain: recent developments. Pain 2002. 96 (3): 221–225.

[10] Mayer EA. Gut feelings: the emerging biology of gut-brain communication. Nature Review Neuroscience 2011. 12 (8): 453–466.

[11] Malykhina AP. Neural mechanisms of pelvic organ cross-sensitization. Neuroscience 2007. 149(3): 660–672.

[12] Grover M, Herfarth H, Drossman DA. The functional-organic dichotomy: postinfectious irritable bowel syndrome and inflammatory bowel disease-irritable bowel syndrome. Clinical Gastroenterology and Hepatology 2009. 7(1): 48–53.

Chapter 2

Psychiatric Comorbidities in Irritable Bowel Syndrome (IBS)

Mihaela Fadgyas Stanculete

Additional information is available at the end of the chapter

http://dx.doi.org/10.5772/66301

Abstract

FA lot of research has pointed out that irritable bowel syndrome (IBS) is a multifactorial illness involving visceral hypersensitivity, alteration of communication between the enteric nervous system (ENS) and central nervous system (CNS), increased intestinal permeability, minimal intestinal inflammation, and altered intestinal microflora. Psychological, social, and genetic factors appear to be important in the development of IBS symptomatology through several mechanisms. This chapter addresses the relationships between irritable bowel syndrome (IBS) and psychiatric comorbidities. The aim of this chapter is to provide an overview of explanatory hypothesis and to describe a variety of approaches which integrate the vast research data about IBS and psychiatric comorbidities, including genetic, brain imaging, and neuropsychological findings. The section of this chapter which overlooks the psychotropic treatment reviews the comparative efficacy of various drugs.

Keywords: irritable bowel syndrome, neuroimaging, psychiatric comorbidities, psychosocial factors

1. Introduction

Irritable bowel syndrome (IBS) is a chronic functional gastrointestinal (GI) disorder that has been reported to be associated with increased use of health-care resources and impaired quality of life.

Over the last two decades, it is becoming increasingly clear that many factors are involved in IBS, and they interact in very complex ways, which have not been yet elucidated.

The biopsychosocial model has been developed to explain the IBS pathogenesis better. According to this model, the gastrointestinal function is modulated via brain-gut axis by psychosocial factors. Particular attention is given to stress, emotion, and psychological factors in the IBS pathogenesis.

Emerging data reveals the interaction between psychiatric disorders and IBS, which suggests that this association should not be ignored when developing strategies for screening and treatment. The simultaneous presence of a mental disorder and IBS worsen the prognosis of both diseases involved to a significantly greater extent.

It is very important to understand better how social and psychological factors influence biological processes both in IBS and psychiatric conditions. Several mechanisms have been proposed to explain this association. In this chapter, we highlight data from a wide range of research including genetic, neurotransmitter, and brain imaging studies.

Stressful life events can lead to the activation of hypothalamic-pituitary-adrenal (HPA) axis. Neurotransmitters including serotonin, norepinephrine, and corticotropin-releasing factor change the motility and the perception in the gut. Brain regions necessary for pain processing and pain and emotional regulation may be involved. The psychological burden of a chronic relapsing illness can increase the maladaptive behaviors and negative emotions and decrease the coping abilities. A better understanding of these processes will be crucial for developing more useful treatments.

Although pharmacological treatments have proven efficacy in IBS, the illness remains chronic with the symptomatic and functional problems only partially influenced for most patients.

A lot of papers have documented improved clinical prognosis in IBS through psychological and pharmacologic interventions. Despite these promising data, the evidence is still limited by underpowered sample sizes.

With this growing awareness of the importance of psychosocial factors in IBS care, medical professionals experience an increased need for accessible background information and practical guidelines for diagnosis and management of psychiatric comorbidities.

Over the last two decades, it is becoming increasingly clear that many factors are involved in IBS and they interact in very complex ways, which have not been yet elucidated.

2. Psychosocial factors linked to IBS

The biopsychosocial model aims to integrate the multidimensional mechanisms to understand how IBS can be developed under such multiple interactions. The most important characteristic of this model is the bidirectional causality: the psychosocial factors influence the brain and the gut, and the gut interacts with the brain via the autonomic nervous system and the hypothalamic-pituitary-adrenal (HPA) axis [1]. The principal psychological and social factors that have been reported to contribute to the onset, the severity, and the evolution of IBS are presented in **Table 1**.

http://dx.doi.org/10.5772/66301

Sociological factors	– Parental beliefs and behaviors – Illness behavior – Learning through positive reinforcement or reward and modeling – Adverse life events (sexual, emotional, physical abuse) – Chronic life stress – Social support – Culture (cultural beliefs, norms)
Psychological factors	– Anxiety, depression – Anger – Cognitive-affective processes: gastrointestinal anxiety, hypervigilance, and attentional bias, catastrophizing, alexithymia – Coping mechanisms

Table 1. Psychological and sociological factors involved in IBS.

- Parental beliefs and behaviors. It is accepted that there is a familial aggregation of IBS. Studies demonstrated that not only the genetic factors could explain why IBS tends to cluster in families, but the development of gastrointestinal symptoms could also be explained by reinforcement and modeling of gastrointestinal illness behavior by parents [2].

- Positive reinforcement of illness behavior. Children whose parents reinforce sickness behavior (through parental protective behaviors) report more severe pain and more school absences than other children. Studies of childhood learning have also suggested that social learning through modeling processes (children observing and learning to exhibit the behaviors they witness) may also contribute to the intergenerational transmission of GI illness behavior and play a significant role in development and maintenance of IBS symptoms [3–5].

- Various types of early adverse life events (EALs) are associated with the development of IBS, in particular sexual, emotional, and physical abuse [6]. The relationship between abuse and severity of gastrointestinal symptoms and poorer health-related quality of life (HRQOL) seems to be partially mediated by concomitant mood disturbances [7]. Studies have shown that other types of EALs have been associated with an increased vulnerability toward developing IBS (parental death, divorce, or separation) [8]. A substantial body of evidence suggests that epigenetic mechanisms play a major role in the causal link between EALs and IBS. Findings from animal models and human studies highlighted the long-term effects of exposure to stress in early life through changes in gene expression [9]. Furthermore, prospective studies have demonstrated that chronic life stress is the most significant predictor of IBS symptom severity over 16 months. Stress has a marked impact on mucosal immune activation, intestinal sensitivity, permeability, secretion, and motility and through various mechanisms can affect the IBS treatment outcomes [10–12].

- Social support is related to many aspects of IBS. It was shown that social support is reduced in chronic illnesses. The association between the quality of social support and the severity of IBS symptoms was mostly investigated. Perceived adequacy of social support appears to have a positive influence on pain possibly through a reduction in stress levels [13]. In contrast, negative social relationship correlates with increased symptom severity.
- Culture. The impact of culture on the perception and description of IBS symptoms is already known. It was emphasized that cultural beliefs, norms, and behaviors should be taken into account when evaluating the IBS presentation and management of the symptoms. Cultural norms could shape the acceptability of expressing symptomatology and the willingness to seek health-care assistance.
- Gastrointestinal-specific anxiety (GSA) represents "the cognitive, affective, and behavioral response stemming from fear of gastrointestinal symptoms, and the context in which these visceral symptoms occur" indicating awareness of and concern about gastrointestinal sensations. It has been suggested that GSA may be more relevant than general anxiety for symptom severity and health outcome and represents a key predictor of IBS diagnosis. Moreover, GSA was found to be associated with the mental component of quality of life, suggesting that GSA is an important endpoint for different interventions [14].
- Hypervigilance. IBS patients selectively attend to gastrointestinal sensations compared to healthy individuals. Some researchers indicated that visceral hypersensitivity is linked with the hypervigilance toward visceral sensations and a tendency to label them negatively [15]. Hypervigilance may reflect poor coping with gastrointestinal-specific anxiety.
- Attentional bias. Studies indicate that attentional bias toward gastrointestinal sensations is exaggerated and could represent a potential factor in IBS development and maintenance. Researchers reported that focusing attention on bodily sensations leads to increased physical symptom complaints and illness behavior.
- Catastrophizing has been defined as a psychological construct characterized by the tendency to have a distorted negative view of health problems and amplify the threat of symptoms. Cross-sectional studies have found that catastrophizing in IBS is associated with increased pain, increased health-care utilization, and increased disability [16].
- Alexithymia is a multidimensional construct defined as an inability in experiencing, expressing, and describing emotions in a verbal manner. Alexithymia can be conceptualized as a deficit in cognitive processing and emotional regulations. IBS patients present higher levels of alexithymia than general population. Also, studies suggest that alexithymia, a stable trait, could be a stronger predictor of IBS severity than GSA, thus implying that impaired affective awareness may weigh in the clinical presentation of IBS [17].
- Anger represents a negative emotional state that has several dimensions: anger experience, anger expression, and anger control. Inhibited anger expression is associated with depression, pain interference, and the frequency of pain behaviors. There are results that higher

http://dx.doi.org/10.5772/66301

levels of trait anger characterize IBS patients when compared to healthy population, and this may be associated with clinical manifestations [18]. Other studies demonstrated that IBS patients appear to have higher levels of anger than a group of patients with organic bowel diseases.

- Coping mechanisms. Studies have begun to focus on the coping mechanisms because these factors influence treatment options, patients' expectations, and treatment outcome. Coping represents the cognitive and behavioral efforts to deal (reduce or tolerate) with a perceived stressful situation. As mentioned above, the coping can influence the outcome of the illness. Therefore the quality of a coping strategy should be evaluated according to with its effect on the outcome. Lazarus has defined two categories of coping from the cognitive perspective: problem focused and emotion focused [19].

Problem-focused strategies strive for resolving the stressful situation or event or altering the source of the stress. It includes strategies such as:

– Problem solving (managing external aspects of the stressor)

– Seeking information or support in handling the situation (instrumental support)

– Accepting responsibility

– Removing oneself from a stressful situation

Emotion-focused coping represents the efforts to regulate the emotions associated with the situation. It involves strategies as:

– Positive reappraisal

– Distancing

– Escape-avoidance

– Seeking social support

Studies showed that in cases of chronic illnesses, the effects of coping are not influenced by the type of problem, or emotion-focus strategies are used but rather if active or avoidant methods are employed. Moreover, in IBS patients, it seems that the presence or absence of depression and/or anxiety influences how they cope with illness. Maladaptive coping and visceral sensitivity appear to be significantly associated with psychological distress, illness perception directly affecting the maladaptive coping.

Phillips et al. evaluated the role of psychosocial factors in predicting the belonging to IBS group and severity of IBS symptoms [20]. They found that four coping strategies (active coping, instrumental support, self-blame, and positive reframing) were best predictors of IBS.

Coping seems to be a relevant factor in mediating the adverse impact of IBS symptomatology on daily activities. Patients' quality of life could be impaired by the lack of adequate social support and by lower coping abilities acquired through social learning during childhood. Also, the impact of IBS symptoms on HRQOL impairment is mediated by dysfunctional attitudes and avoidant-oriented coping. Inefficient coping strategies represent important treatment targets for cognitive-behavioral therapy (CBT) because coping styles are modulated by the use of cognitive abilities [21].

3. Genes and IBS

As discussed before, IBS is a chronic disease characterized by familial clustering. In the recent years, the hypothesis of a genetic contribution to the development of IBS has gained some support [22].

It was postulated that IBS is a multifactorial, polygenic complex disorder. A candidate gene study evaluates a specific polymorphism or set of polymorphisms. Until now, approximately 60 candidate genes were investigated to determine whether specific genetic variants may be associated with IBS. Until now the data sustaining the genetic hypothesis are scarce, and some results have not been replicated.

Many epidemiological studies reported psychiatric comorbidities, and also reported higher rates of these comorbidities than in the general population. Different pathways could be affected in the subgroup of IBS patients with psychiatric comorbidities. Recent studies tried to evaluate if the IBS and mental disorders share common genetic pathways (primary corticotropin-releasing system and serotoninergic pathway).

Data are sustaining that HPA axis and serotoninergic system are likely to be involved in the genetic susceptibility to major depressive disorder, but currently, there is no clinical evidence for a common gene in IBS and major depression.

Eight genes involved in psychiatric disorders were investigated with mixed results:

1. FKBP5 gene (the gene encoding FK506-binding protein 51) is located on the short arm of chromosome 5; some variants were associated with stress reactivity and post-traumatic stress disorder (PTSD) risk.

2. Catechol-O-methyltransferase (COMT) gene: COMT Val158Met was related to IBS with constipation. The same variant was associated with obsessive-compulsive disorder (OCD), panic disorder (PD), and cognitive performance.

3. Opioid receptor Mu 1 (OPRM1) gene: diseases related to this gene include opioid dependence, pain sensitivity, and social sensitivity. OPRM1 118AG variant was associated with IBS-mixed and IBS-diarrhea (IBS-D).

4. Brain-derived neurotrophic factor (BDNF) gene: psychiatric diseases related to this gene include schizophrenia, anorexia and bulimia nervosa, PTSD, and mood disorders. BDNF Val166Met was associated with IBS with psychiatric comorbidities.

5. Neuropeptide Y (NPY) gene is implicated in stress response

6. Ankyrin repeat and kinase domain containing 1 (ANKK1) gene: it was associated with impulse control disorders and alexithymia.

http://dx.doi.org/10.5772/66301

7. Dopamine receptor D2 (DRD2) gene: it seems to have a role in cocaine dependence.

8. Fatty acid amide hydrolase (FAAH) gene also has a role in substance dependence.

A recent study found preliminary evidence that IBS patients with comorbid anxiety or depression are more likely to present functional variant alleles of serotonin transporters than IBS patients without psychiatric comorbidities.

Maybe the new technological advances in genomic studies will make it possible to identify common and rare variants on genomic deoxyribonucleic acid (DNA) [23]. Until now, based on candidate gene studies, it appears that there may be a different molecular basis for IBS with comorbid anxiety versus IBS without comorbid anxiety. Thus the role of environmental factor contributors to IBS development should not be underestimated.

4. Psychiatric comorbidity in IBS

Many studies reported an increased frequency of psychiatric comorbidities (diagnosis and symptoms) among patients with IBS. It has been estimated that IBS patients have high rates of psychiatric comorbidities (50 %–90 %). There are multiple factors involved in the determination of this comorbidity. The latest disease models of IBS encompass the overlap of brain circuits involved in emotion regulation, autonomic responses, and pain modulation as the most important features.

Clinical reports indicate that the relationship between IBS and psychiatric illnesses is bidirectional between the gastrointestinal tract and the brain, through various pathways (neural, neuroimmune, and neuroendocrine). Among mental disorders, mood disorders, anxiety disorders, and somatoform disorders have been the most frequently diagnosed conditions [24]. The complexity of the underlying pathophysiological processes is not completely understood. The hypothesis linking cognitive and emotional areas in the central nervous system (CNS) with the autonomic nervous system (ANS) and the enteric system (ENS) had a significant contribution to the understanding of the pathogenesis of IBS.

The increased comorbidity among IBS and psychiatric disorders is well established. Even though data refers to patients seen in tertiary gastroenterology centers, recent data pointed out that psychiatric comorbidity is also present in primary care.

Another important aspect that should be emphasized is that the majority of the study results are based on the administration of self-report screening instruments rather than a psychiatric interview. The screening tools only assess the probability of a psychiatric diagnosis, but further investigations are necessary. Moreover, studies of a causal relationship between IBS and psychiatric comorbidities are still limited in number and provide contradictory data.

Some authors argued that the data are applying only to those patients who have sought treatment and are not applicable to the non-consulters. Others suggested that could be a subset of patients with IBS characterized by high psychiatric comorbidity. Nevertheless, there is some evidence supporting the biological association between IBS and mental disorders.

Approximately 50 % of patients with a psychiatric disorder develop the disease before the GI symptoms became manifest, and psychiatric symptoms appear to develop at the same time in a majority of the remaining 50 %.

Many studies pointed out that worry-rumination can influence the brain-gut axis. Moreover, it has been identified as one fundamental factor that mediates the high co-occurrence of the two most frequent psychiatric comorbidities in IBS patients (anxiety and depression) [25].

It is noteworthy that the patients with severe IBS and comorbid psychiatric disorders have been found to have a higher impairment in HRQOL, elevated symptom burden, increased functional disability, and increased health-care costs.

4.1. Mood disorders and IBS

Many studies have investigated the prevalence of depression among IBS patients, but the results are vastly variable, ranging from high to much lower rates. There are also studies showing that patients with major depressive disorders present gastrointestinal symptoms.

Relevant findings from a large-scale population-based study suggest that depression and stress are independent risk factors for IBS. In this study, the incidence rate of IBS was higher in the patients with mild depression than in those with severe depression.

Several authors reported that IBS is associated with suicidality. The findings of one study indicate that 4 % of IBS patients who sought help from primary care, 16 % from secondary care, and 38 % from tertiary care endorsed suicidal ideation determined primary by the gastrointestinal symptoms. A systematic review indicated that IBS patients were two to four times more likely to recognize a history of suicidal behavior, even in the absence of depression.

A study conducted by Guthrie et al. revealed three definite groups of IBS patients [26]:

- Distressed high utilizers: characterized by multiple psychosocial comorbidities, increase levels of health-care utilization, high frequency of sexual abuse, and low pain thresholds to rectal balloon distension; the patients from this group reported suicidal ideation and self-harm history.
- Distressed low utilizers: marked by high psychiatric comorbidity, low physician consultations, low frequency of sexual abuse, and low pain threshold.
- Tolerant low utilizers: characterized by low rates of psychiatric comorbidities, low levels of consultations, and high pain thresholds.

It should be taken into account that an increase in suicidal ideation is not entirely explained by the symptom intensity and the presence of anxiety or depressive comorbidity. Therefore, IBS patients, especially distressed high utilizers, should be assessed for suicidality [27].

4.2. Anxiety disorders and IBS

As mentioned earlier, there is a higher prevalence of anxiety disorders among IBS patients than in the general population (47 % versus 26 %). According to the available literature, the most prevalent anxiety disorders among patients with IBS are generalized anxiety disorder (GAD) and panic disorder (PD). Some studies suggest that mixed IBS (IBS-M) patients are more likely to present higher scores for anxiety, especially in comparison with IBS with constipation (IBS-C) [25].

It must be noted that recent studies suggest that the strong association between GAD morbidity and IBS observed in tertiary centers was not a consequence of increased help-seeking behavior.

PD and IBS share common characteristics such as gastrointestinal symptoms, anticipatory anxiety, and avoidant behavior because of fear of symptoms. Based on results of different studies, it appears that the presence of IBS is associated with greater severity of agoraphobia, anticipatory anxiety, and panic attacks in PD patients. Moreover, patients with IBS reported having high scores of anxiety sensitivity, as the PD patients. Further information on IBS and PD came from a review emphasizing that the experience of feeling uncontrollable somatic symptoms, very common in IBS, could be a stimulating component for PD in patients with subclinical PD symptoms [28].

4.3. Somatoform disorders and IBS

IBS is considered a functional disorder, and it is congruent with the definition of somatoform disorders. The Diagnostic and Statistical Manual for Mental Disorders (DSM-4-TR) and the International Classification of Diseases (ICD) classify physical symptoms that cannot be medically explained together with persistent requests for medical investigations in a separate somatoform category. In the DSM-5 this category was renamed as "somatic symptoms disorder" (SSD) and redefined; there is no longer a demand for lack of "medical" explanation of symptoms. It means that this diagnosis could be a primary diagnosis (somatic symptoms may be medically unexplained) or could be a secondary diagnosis in patients who have an organic illness. The documented prevalence rates of somatoform disorders among IBS patients vary from 15 % to 48 % [29].

5. Neuroimaging in IBS

Studies using structural and functional techniques in IBS patients showed abnormalities that were associated with:

- Visceral hypersensitivity
- Impairment of affective processes involved in visceral pain modulation
- Alteration of descending pain inhibitory pathways

Data obtained from brain imaging studies in IBS demonstrated physiological differences that distinguish patients with IBS from a healthy population. The results obtained have varied maybe because of different study designs or due to the heterogeneity of study populations [30, 31].

5.1. Structural neuroimaging

Nowadays, structural approaches are provided mainly by diffusion tensor imaging (DTI) and by structural magnetic resonance imaging (sMRI). The studies focus on structural connectivity.

IBS patients with chronic pain have regional cortical thickness (CT) alterations in comparison with healthy controls. CT represents the results of neural reorganization of pain circuits and regions associated with sensorial processing.

IBS patients present decreased gray matter density in prefrontal and parietal regions and in emotional circuits. Ellingson et al. demonstrated in a study using DTI that IBS patients have microstructural changes in areas involved in the cortical pain modulatory areas and cortico-thalamic modulation. The anterior insula and basal ganglia (BS) have a prominent role in the integration of sensory and non-sensory information.

Another study demonstrated that IBS patients showed lower cortical thickness (CT) in the interoceptive association cortex (aINS) in the right hemisphere than in healthy controls.

The anterior insular subregion has multiple roles:

- Integration of food-related (olfaction and taste), interoceptive, emotional, and cognitive functions
- Provides output to autonomic and pain modulation systems
- Plays a key role in prediction, error processing, and self-awareness of sensations

In the relationship with these roles, insular regions seem to be involved in psychopathology. As already highlighted, patients with IBS have an abnormal processing of visceral pain in this area as a result of the dysfunctional inhibition of the pain in cortical areas. Patients reporting higher levels of pain intensity associated with their IBS symptoms presented an important CT in the bilateral orbitofrontal cortex (OFC). Also, it was observed that disease duration and pain intensity were correlated with CT in the dorsolateral prefrontal cortex (DLPFC) and OFC, bilaterally.

Other studies reported CT in the anterior midcingulate cortex (aMCC), ventrolateral prefrontal cortex (vlPFC), and thalamus. The structural changes of gray matter density in the periaqueductal gray (PAG) region may be a reflection of the compromised descending modulation of pain.

Blankstein evidenced increased gray matter density in the hypothalamus of the IBS patients.

Depression and anxiety have a well-established role in the modulation of pain. It was suggested that the decreased gray matter density in the anterior/medial thalamus in patients with IBS could be related to the clinical levels of anxiety or depression.

Interestingly, some authors suggested that structural changes in the primary interoceptive cortex, as well as in the attentional and emotional network, could represent endophenotypes of IBS.

http://dx.doi.org/10.5772/66301

5.2. Functional neuroimaging

Functional approaches are provided by single-positron emission computerized tomography (SPECT), positron emission tomography (PET), resting-state magnetic resonance (MRI) and functional magnetic resonance (fMRI), magnetic resonance spectroscopy (MRS), near-infrared spectroscopic imaging (NIRSI), and magnetoencephalography (MEG).

A recent meta-analysis of research on cortical responses to rectal distension suggests the conclusion that brain responses to rectal distension are different in IBS patients and healthy controls. IBS patients showed greater activation in brain regions involved in emotional processing, cognitive modulation, and interoceptive analysis.

Using the functional neuroimaging techniques in IBS patients, it was identified the hyperactivity of the amygdala (an essential component in the emotional arousal network). The amygdala network is involved in processing visceral input in relation to emotional stimuli, modulation of sensorial information, and emotional regulation.

Another area that exhibited functional alteration during experimental pain in IBS patients is represented by the basal ganglia (BG). The data obtained are consistent with the reduction of the dendritic density in cortico-basal ganglia-thalamic-cortical circuits involved in modulation of pain. Moreover, hypersensitive IBS patients present more DLPFC activation than normosensitive patients.

The results obtained in studies using neuroimaging techniques sustain the hypothesis that IBS have a biological substrate, but the same changes could be noticed in other chronic disorders. Furthermore, psychosocial factors (early-life trauma, catastrophizing, anxiety, and depression) have had a substantial impact on the neuroimaging correlations of IBS. An association was noticed (either positive or negative) between the level of psychopathology and neuroimaging findings, thus emphasizing the relevance of psychological factors in IBS determinism [32–34].

6. Neuropsychological findings in IBS

Stress induces changes in HPA axis functioning with neurobiological and cognitive consequences. The brain-gut axis appears to have a major importance of cognitive performance. The psychiatric comorbidity has also impact in the neurocognitive functioning [15, 35].

In general, normal cognitive functioning was reported in IBS, but some researchers demonstrated subtle cognitive deficits that remained after the correction for psychiatric comorbidity.

6.1. Attention and IBS

Attention is a behavioral and cognitive process involving the selection of sensory information to optimize current behavioral responses to specific stimuli relevant for the organism.

Researchers suggest that IBS patients have specific abnormalities in attentional network functioning. IBS patients present attentional biases for pain words. Attentional alterations are associated with increased pain report and illness behavior.

6.2. Memory and IBS

Currently, there are data suggesting impairment in visuospatial memory in patients with IBS. The researchers found that IBS patients displayed poorer performance in hippocampal-mediated visuospatial tasks than non-IBS controls. They made twice to three times as many errors on the visuospatial test as the healthy control group. It was suggested that visuospatial memory dysfunction could represent a common component of IBS [36].

6.3. Executive function and IBS

Cognitive flexibility in IBS patients was evaluated with Wisconsin Card Sorting Test (WCST). Recent researches have shown that IBS patients present latent impairments in the cognitive flexibility. The biological substrate for those findings seems to be the modified activity of the DLPFC, hippocampus, and insula. Also, the altered connectivity between the DLPFC and pre-supplementary motor area appears to be involved [37].

7. Psychopharmacology of IBS

Treatment of IBS could be classified in pharmacologic and non-pharmacological strategies. The choice of therapy depends on types of symptoms and their severity and frequency. It is clear that many aspects of IBS may be linked to psychosocial stressors and psychiatric comorbidities. More recent research emphasized that the psychotropic drugs can play a major role in the treatment of IBS patients [38].

7.1. Antidepressants

IBS is characterized by abnormalities in visceral sensations and dysregulation of central pain perception. Thus, the antidepressants represent a treatment option in patients with moderate and severe symptoms. The antidepressants were found to be efficacious for abdominal pain but have no effect on bowel habit. Moreover, their tolerance may represent a problem. Currently, antidepressants are used as a second-line therapy. The beneficial effects of antidepressants could be the results of influence in central pain threshold (an increase of threshold). Other mechanisms of action are represented by the anticholinergic effects (influence on gastrointestinal motility and secretion) and by reducing the pain sensitivity of peripheral nerves [39].

7.1.1. Tricyclics antidepressants (TCA)

Most recent research supports the use of TCAs in IBS treatment. The effects of several TCAs including clomipramine, nortriptyline, and imipramine were investigated in IBS patients. The results showed that the required dose of TCAs is lower than that used to treat patients with depression. TCAs are effective in IBS-D due to the prolongment of whole-gut transit times. A systematic review of 11 randomized controlled trials RCTs comparing TCAs and placebo revealed that the benefit attributable to TCA therapy relative to placebo was 12.5 %. The

http://dx.doi.org/10.5772/66301

numbers needed to treat (NNT) were four, equal or superior to other pharmacological agents (like motility agents and probiotics). The TCAs slow gut-transit time and could be used in diarrhea-predominant IBS.

7.1.2. Selective serotonin reuptake inhibitors (SSRIs)

Efficacy of SSRIs in the treatment of IBS was evaluated in seven randomized trials comparing SSRIs with placebo. The SSRIs studied were fluoxetine, paroxetine, and citalopram. One small open trial demonstrated the efficacy of paroxetine on abdominal pain. A common limitation of all the studies is represented by the short duration of the study (12 weeks) and the small sample size. The relative risks (RR) in the treatment of IBS symptoms were 0.62, but significant heterogeneity characterized the studies. The SSRIs decrease orocecal transit and would be of greater benefit in constipation-predominant IBS. According to Cochrane database of systematic reviews, SSRIs are prescribed at dosages standard for treating psychiatric disorders and should be used as a third-line treatment.

7.1.3. Serotonin-noradrenaline reuptake inhibitors (SNRIs)

Both serotonin and norepinephrine have a role in visceral motility and visceral sensation. It was noticed that low-dose SNRIs (duloxetine and venlafaxine) seem to be more efficacious than SSRIs. One study performed on healthy volunteers showed that venlafaxine reduced pain sensation ratings in response to grade distensions but did not have a significant impact on the colonic transit. SNRIs are promising, but more studies need to be done.

7.2. Atypical antipsychotics

Quetiapine may help patients with IBS by decreasing the anxiety and ameliorating sleep disturbances. It also augments the effect of antidepressants and provides an independent analgesic effect [40].

7.3. Anticonvulsants

Preliminary data from animal models provides evidence suggesting that the γ-aminobutyric acidergic (GABA) agents (gabapentin) and $\alpha 2\delta$ ligand (pregabalin) may also be efficient in reducing central sensitization in hyperalgesia [41]. Gabapentin has more recently been used in the treatment of chronic pain. Pregabalin has been shown to be more potent than gabapentin. In patients with IBS, both gabapentin and pregabalin have been shown to reduce rectal sensitivity to balloon distension, but currently, there are no results published from clinical trials examining the efficacy of $\alpha 2\delta$ ligands on symptoms in IBS patients.

7.4. Anxiolytic agents

The rationale for the use of anxiolytic drugs for the treatment of IBS likely came from the observation that the majority of patients also present of comorbid anxiety. Buspirone, an azapirone, is an anti-anxiolytic nonbenzodiazepine drug. It is a partial serotonin 1A (5-HT1A) receptor agonist used to augment the effects of antidepressants. The effects on gastrointestinal motility are represented by the reduction of funding tone and the delay of emptying. Also, a relaxation effect on the rectal tone was observed [42].

8. Conclusions

There is a general agreement that a global assessment of IBS patient should be done. The significant overlap between IBS and mental disorders should encourage the clinicians to evaluate for comorbid psychiatric disorders routinely. It is very important to recognize the linkage between psychiatric diagnoses and IBS because these comorbid conditions are characterized by increased symptom burden and additive functional impairment. Thus, successful management of patients with IBS requires careful attention to all psychosocial factors involved.

Author details

Mihaela Fadgyas Stanculete[1,2*]

Address all correspondence to: mihaelastanculete@yahoo.com

1 Department of Neurosciences, Discipline of Psychiatry and Pediatric Psychiatry, University of Medicine and Pharmacy "Iuliu Hațieganu", Cluj-Napoca, Romania

2 Second Psychiatric Clinic, Emergency County Hospital Cluj, Cluj-Napoca, Romania

References

[1] Tanaka Y, Kanazawa M, Fukudo S, Drossman DA. Biopsychosocial model of irritable bowel syndrome. J Neurogastroenterol Motil. 2011;2:131–9. DOI: 10.5056/jnm.2011.17.2.131

[2] Levy RL, Whitehead WE, Walker LS, Von Korff M, Feld AD, et al. Increased somatic complaints and health-care utilization in children: effects of parent IBS status and parent response to gastrointestinal symptoms. Am J Gastroenterol. 2004;99(12):2442–51. DOI: 10.1111/j.1572-0241.2004.40478.x

[3] Van Oudenhove L, Levy RL, Crowell MD, Drossman DA, Halpert AD, Keefer L, Lackner JM, Murphy TB, Naliboff BD. Biopsychosocial aspects of functional gastrointestinal disorders: how central and environmental processes contribute to the development and expression of functional gastrointestinal disorders. Gastroenterology. 2016;150(6):1355–67. DOI: http://dx.doi.org/10.1053/j.gastro.2016.02.027

[4] Vervoort T, Huguet A, Verhoeven K, Goubert L. Mothers' and fathers' responses to their child's pain moderate the relationship between the child's pain catastrophizing and disability. PAIN®. 2011;152(4):786–93. DOI: 10.1016/j.pain.2010.12.010

[5] Van Tilburg MA, Levy RL, Walker LS, Von Korff M, Feld LD, Garner M, Feld AD, Whitehead WE. Psychosocial mechanisms for the transmission of somatic symptoms from parents to children. WJG. 2015;21(18):5532. DOI: 10.3748/wjg.v21.i18.5532.

[6] Bradford K, Shih W, Videlock EJ, Presson AP, Naliboff BD, Mayer EA, Chang L. Association between early adverse life events and irritable bowel syndrome. Clin Gastroenterol Hepatol. 2012;10(4):385–90. DOI: 10.1016/j.cgh.2011.12.018

[7] Drossman DA. Abuse, trauma, and GI illness: is there a link?. Am J Gastroenterol. 2011;106(1):14–25. DOI: 10.1038/ajg.2010.453

[8] Chitkara DK, van Tilburg MA, Blois-Martin N, Whitehead WE. Early life risk factors that contribute to irritable bowel syndrome in adults: a systematic review. Am J Gastroenterol. 2008;103(3):765–74. DOI: 10.1111/j.1572-0241.2007.01722.x

[9] O'Mahony SM, Hyland NP, Dinan TG, Cryan JF. Maternal separation as a model of brain–gut axis dysfunction. Psychopharmacology. 2011;214(1):71–88. DOI: 10.1007/s00213-010-2010-9

[10] Moloney RD, Johnson AC, O'Mahony SM, Dinan TG, Meerveld GV, Cryan JF. Stress and the microbiota–gut–brain axis in visceral pain: relevance to irritable bowel syndrome. CNS Neurosci Ther. 2016;22(2):102–17. DOI: 10.1111/cns.12490

[11] Vanuytsel T, van Wanrooy S, Vanheel H, Vanormelingen C, Verschueren S, Houben E, Rasoel SS, Tóth J, Holvoet L, Farré R, Van Oudenhove L. Psychological stress and corticotropin-releasing hormone increase intestinal permeability in humans by a mast cell-dependent mechanism. Gut. 2014;63(8):1293–9. DOI: 10.1136/gutjnl-2013-305690

[12] Van Oudenhove L, Aziz Q. Recent insights on central processing and psychological processes in functional gastrointestinal disorders. Dig Liv Dis. 2009;41(11):781–7. DOI: 10.1016/j.dld.2009.07.004

[13] Lackner JM, Brasel AM, Quigley BM, Keefer L, Krasner SS, Powell C, Katz LA, Sitrin MD. The ties that bind: perceived social support, stress, and IBS in severely affected patients. Neurogastroenterol Motil. 2010;22(8):893–900. DOI: 10.1111/j.1365-2982.2010.01516.x

[14] Jerndal P, Ringström G, Agerforz P, Karpefors M, Akkermans LM, Bayati A, Simrén M. Gastrointestinal-specific anxiety: an important factor for severity of GI symptoms and

quality of life in IBS. Neurogastroenterol Motil. 2010;22(6):646-e179. DOI: 10.1111/j. 1365-2982.2010.01493

[15] Kennedy PJ, Clarke G, Quigley EM, Groeger JA, Dinan TG, Cryan JF. Gut memories: towards a cognitive neurobiology of irritable bowel syndrome. Neurosci Biobehav Rev. 2012;36(1):310–40. DOI: 10.1016/j.neubiorev.2011.07.001

[16] Hunt MG, Milonova M, Moshier S. Catastrophizing the consequences of gastrointestinal symptoms in irritable bowel syndrome. J Cogn Psychother. 2009;23(2):160–73. DOI: 10.1891/0889-8391.23.2.160

[17] Porcelli P, De Carne M, Leandro G. Alexithymia and gastrointestinal-specific anxiety in moderate to severe irritable bowel syndrome. Compr Psych. 2014;55(7):1647–53. DOI: 10.1016/j.comppsych.2014.05.022

[18] Fadgyas Stănculete M, Pojoga C, Dumitrascu DL. Experience of anger in patients with irritable bowel syndrome in Romania. Clujul Medical. 2014;87(2):98. DOI: 10.15386/ cjmed-290

[19] Lazarus RS. Coping theory and research: past, present, and future. Psychosom Med. 1993;55(3):234–47.

[20] Phillips K, Wright BJ, Kent S. Psychosocial predictors of irritable bowel syndrome diagnosis and symptom severity. J Psychosom Res. 2013;75(5):467–74. DOI: 10.1016/ j.jpsychores.2013.08.002.

[21] Grodzinsky E, Walter S, Viktorsson L, Carlsson AK, Jones MP, Faresjö Å. More negative self-esteem and inferior coping strategies among patients diagnosed with IBS compared with patients without IBS-a case–control study in primary care. BMC Fam Pract. 2015;16(1):1. DOI: 10.1186/s12875-015-0225-x

[22] Saito YA. The role of genetics in IBS. Gastroenterol Clin North Am. 2011;40(1):45–67. DOI: 10.1016/j.gtc.2010.12.011

[23] Henström M, D'Amato M. Genetics of irritable bowel syndrome. Mol Cell Pediatr. 2016;3(1):1. DOI: 10.1186/s40348-016-0038-6

[24] Garakani A, Win T, Virk S, Gupta S, Kaplan D, Masand PS. Comorbidity of irritable bowel syndrome in psychiatric patients: a review. Am J Ther. 2003;10(1):61–7. DOI: 10.1097/00045391-200301000-00014

[25] Fond G, Loundou A, Hamdani N, Boukouaci W, Dargel A, Oliveira J, Roger M, Tamouza R, Leboyer M, Boyer L. Anxiety and depression comorbidities in irritable bowel syndrome (IBS): a systematic review and meta-analysis. Eur Arch Psychiatry Clin Neurosci. 2014;264(8):651–60. DOI: 10.1007/s00406-014-0502-z

[26] Guthrie E, Barlow J, Fernandes L, Ratcliffe J, Read N, Thompson DG, Tomenson B, Creed F, North of England IBS Research Group. Changes in tolerance to rectal distension correlate with changes in psychological state in patients with severe

irritable bowel syndrome. Psychosom Med. 2004;66(4):578–82. DOI: 10.1097/01.psy.0000128899.22514.c0

[27] Spiegel BM. The burden of IBS: looking at metrics. Curr Gastroenterol Rep. 2009;11(4):265–9. DOI: 10.1007/s11894-009-0039-x

[28] Hausteiner-Wiehle C, Henningsen P. Irritable bowel syndrome: relations with functional, mental, and somatoform disorders. World J Gastroenterol WJG. 2014;20(20):6024–30. DOI: 10.3748/wjg.v20.i20.60240.6024

[29] Wouters MM, Boeckxstaens GE. Is there a causal link between psychological disorders and functional gastrointestinal disorders?. Expert Rev Gastroenterol Hepatol. 2016;10(1):5–8. DOI: 10.1586/17474124.2016.1109446

[30] Weaver KR, Sherwin LB, Walitt B, Melkus GD, Henderson WA. Neuroimaging the brain-gut axis in patients with irritable bowel syndrome. WJGPT. 2016;7(2):320–33. DOI: 10.4292/WJGPT.v7.i2.320

[31] Beauregard M. Mind does really matter: evidence from neuroimaging studies of emotional self-regulation, psychotherapy, and placebo effect. Prog Neurobiol. 2007;81(4):218–36.DOI: 10.1016/j.pneurobio.2007.01.005

[32] Mayer EA, Labus JS, Tillisch K, Cole SW, Baldi P. Towards a systems view of IBS. Nat Rev Gastroenterol Hepatol. 2015;12(10):592–605. DOI: 10.1038/nrgastro.2015.121

[33] Ma X, Li S, Tian J, Jiang G, Wen H, Wang T, Fang J, Zhan W, Xu Y. Altered brain spontaneous activity and connectivity network in irritable bowel syndrome patients: a resting-state fMRI study. Clin Neurophysiol. 2015;126(6):1190–7. DOI: 10.1016/j.clinph.2014.10.004

[34] Blankstein U, Chen J, Diamant NE, Davis KD. Altered brain structure in irritable bowel syndrome: potential contributions of pre-existing and disease-driven factors. Gastroenterology. 2010;138(5):1783–9. DOI: 10.1053/j.gastro.2009.12.043

[35] Attree EA, Dancey CP, Keeling D, Wilson C. Cognitive function in people with chronic illness: inflammatory bowel disease and irritable bowel syndrome. Appl Neuropsychol. 2003;10(2):96–104. DOI: 10.1207/S15324826AN1002_05

[36] Kennedy PJ, Clarke G, O'Neill A, Groeger JA, Quigley EM, Shanahan F, Cryan JF, Dinan TG. Cognitive performance in irritable bowel syndrome: evidence of a stress-related impairment in visuospatial memory. Psychol Med. 2014;44(07):1553–66. DOI: 10.1017/S0033291713002171

[37] Aizawa E, Sato Y, Kochiyama T, Saito N, Izumiyama M, Morishita J, Kanazawa M, Shima K, Mushiake H, Hongo M, Fukudo S. Altered cognitive function of prefrontal cortex during error feedback in patients with irritable bowel syndrome, based on FMRI

and dynamic causal modeling. Gastroenterology. 2012;143(5):1188–98. DOI: 10.1053/j.gastro.2012.07.104

[38] Sinagra E, Romano C, Cottone M. Psychopharmacological treatment and psychological interventions in irritable bowel syndrome. Gastroenterol Res Pract. 2012;2012:486067. DOI: 10.1155/2012/486067

[39] Ruepert L, Quartero AO, de Wit NJ, van der Heijden GJ, Rubin G, Muris JW. Bulking agents, antispasmodics and antidepressants for the treatment of irritable bowel syndrome. Cochrane Datbase Syst Rev. 2011. DOI: 10.1002/14651858.CD003460.pub3

[40] Halland M, Talley NJ. New treatments for IBS. Nat Rev Gastroenterol Hepatol. 2013;10(1):13–23. DOI: 10.1038/nrgastro.2012.207

[41] Lee KJ, Kim JH, Cho SW. Gabapentin reduces rectal mechanosensitivity and increases rectal compliance in patients with diarrhoea-predominant irritable bowel syndrome. Aliment Pharmacol Ther. 2005;22(10):981–8. DOI: 10.1111/j.1365-2036.2005.02685.x

[42] O'Mahony S, Chua AS, Quigley EM, Clarke G, Shanahan F, Keeling PW, Dinan TG. Evidence of an enhanced central 5HT response in irritable bowel syndrome and in the rat maternal separation model. Neurogastroenterol Motil. 2008;20(6):680–8. DOI: 10.1111/j.1365-2982.2007.01065.x

Chapter 3

Inflammation as a Potential Therapeutic Target in IBS

Alexandra Chira, Romeo Ioan Chira and
Dan Lucian Dumitrascu

Additional information is available at the end of the chapter

http://dx.doi.org/10.5772/66193

Abstract

The pathogenesis of irritable bowel syndrome (IBS) has been intensively researched, and despite a long journey for unraveling all the structures and the pathways involved, it still remains partially obscure. Inflammation was the first to be hypothesized as a potential pathway for the pathogenesis of IBS. It remains a keystone in the complex machinery of the pathogenesis that is currently considered multifactorial. Elucidating the pathogenesis of IBS is crucial for a targeted therapy of the disease. In this chapter, we review information regarding gut inflammation in IBS, underlining some of the newest data or the cornerstones. Additionally, our aim was also to review treatment currently available and future perspectives regarding anti-inflammatory treatments for IBS. Newer techniques allow detection and research of mediators involved in inflammation, as well as their potential role to be targeted by pharmacological agents. Recent data supports not only further research of the newer agents that are currently being developed but also some of the available ones that do not have sufficient evidence. Emerging therapies that target inflammation are under evaluation, in trials. A multidrug or a multidisciplinary approach needs to be considered in some cases that fail to respond to current treatment.

Keywords: anti-inflammatory, inflammation, irritable bowel syndrome, IBS treatment, postinfectious

1. Introduction

Despite the intensive research on irritable bowel syndrome (IBS) is being conducted, the pathogenesis still remains partially obscure. Since the description of this syndrome, many researchers have questioned the cause of IBS, which is currently being considered as multifactorial [1–3] with increasing evidence that support the concept [4, 5], since there are multiple mechanisms that could trigger the clinical complaints.

Not just one structure or system is involved in the occurrence of IBS, and there is a complex network already described and currently referred to as brain-gut axis [6–9] with multiple directions and ways to communicate or interrelate between these structures and paths [10] that are reflected also in the heterogeneity of the subtypes of IBS.

Although IBS is a functional gastrointestinal disorder [11] with no structural or biochemical abnormalities, there is some evidence suggesting that in some subtypes of IBS, inflammation might play a key role in generating a low-grade inflammatory response and a spectrum of symptoms that sometimes overlap with those of inflammatory bowel diseases in remission [12, 13], leading to difficulties in establishing the diagnosis in clinical practice.

In this chapter, we will review literature data concerning inflammation and its relation to IBS underlining some of the newest data or the key ones. Our aim was also to review treatment currently available and future perspectives regarding anti-inflammatory treatments for IBS.

2. Inflammation in IBS

Inflammation, defined as the answer of the immune system to various triggers, was first described by Celsus [14], who has assigned to it the four signs: *dolor* (pain), *rubor* (redness), *tumor* (swelling), *calor* (heat), and to which Rudolf Virchow [15] added *functio laesa* (functional impairment). All the characteristics that define inflammation are induced by a complex set of mediators [16]. In addition, the triggers that could initiate inflammatory responses are numerous and diverse [17]. The inflammatory responses may be acute or chronic [16, 17].

Inflammation was one of the first hypothesised causes of IBS [18]. Intestinal inflammation was proposed as a potential mechanism involved in the pathogenesis of IBS since 1960s, when Hiatt et al. [18] described mast cells in the muscularis externa of the terminal colon and cecum. Discovered by Paul Ehrlich, mast cells are the precursors of CD34+ hematopoietic stem cells [19]. Due to the diversity of functions of mast cells, they have been a cornerstone in the study of multiple conditions, being intensively researched in the last decades. Mast cells have multiple functions [20], some of them involving the gut: neuroimmune interactions, epithelial secretion and permeability, and visceral sensation [20, 21]. In addition, it can express receptors for several cytokines that are involved in immunity [19] or release key mediators [22]. Numerous studies assessed the presence and/or the role of mast cells in IBS [23–25]. There are also rigorous papers that reviewed studies investigating mast cells and/or the mast cell mediators in IBS [26].

Other types of mediators, such as immunoglobulin (Ig) E and atopia, have been investigated in IBS and linked to mast cells [27, 28]. Degranulation of mast cells and, subsequently, the release of mast cell mediators can also be induced by IgE [28]. There are few data regarding IgE levels in IBS. Vara et al. [29] showed higher levels of IgE in IBS compared with healthy controls.

http://dx.doi.org/10.5772/66193

Besides mast cells, there are data indicating that inflammatory cells are present in colonic mucosa in IBS patients [23]. They showed on colonic biopsies multiple types of cells such as neutrophils and T lymphocytes besides mast cells, all of which may support the role of the immune system in the ethiopathogenesis of IBS [23, 30]. If most of the studies examined mucosa of the rectum [31, 32], there are few studies that assessed also the deeper layers of the enteral wall [33]. There is a complex local response when triggers are detected [16, 34].

The balance of pro-inflammatory and anti-inflammatory responses and the mediators that are involved in the complex interactions have also been the subject of many studies. There is evidence of sustained inflammation in IBS supported by numerous studies that have detected low anti-inflammatory cytokines in IBS patients [35] or others that found high levels of those pro-inflammatory ones or a misbalance of the pro- and anti-inflammatory cytokine proportion [36, 37]. The complex dialogue between the structures involved in maintaining the homeostasis includes interrelation of nervous, immune, and endocrine systems [30, 34], where a pivotal piece is the brain that governs the humoral and neurological systems [34, 38, 39], in a complex network with multidirectional communicating systems [10]. Not only the anatomical integrity but also the functional status of all the systems is of major importance [40].

Psychological factors can participate in this mechanism, maintaining a state of low inflammation [41]. Inflammation in the gut might be responsible also for hyperalgesia [42] present in some patients with IBS contributing to the maintenance of the complaints.

2.1. Postinfectious IBS

Postinfectious IBS (PI-IBS) is a more recently coined type of IBS, initially identified as post-dysenteric IBS (PD-IBS) [43]. PI-IBS is defined as a subset of IBS in which the onset of IBS symptoms develops after an infectious episode and was first described by Chaudhary and Truelove [43]. This entity was confirmed by other studies [44]. The incidence of PI-IBS varies between 4 and 32% [45–47]. More frequently, PI-IBS was described and studied after an enteral infection [44, 48]. Pathogens already recognized to be involved in enteral infections are the following:

- bacteria: *Campylobacter jejuni* [31], *Salmonella enterica* [45], *Shigella* [49], *Escherichia coli* [50–52], *Clostridium difficile* [53]
- viruses: *Norovirus* [50, 54]
- parasites: *Giardia lamblia* [50, 55], *Blastocystis* spp. [56], *Dientamoeba fragilis* [57]

This subset of IBS patients offers a strong support emphasizing the importance of inflammation as one of the main paths to IBS. Enteral pathogens may induce pathological changes [31]. Spiller et al. [31] reported an imbalance of the enteroendocrine cells and of T lymphocytes, these two being assessed by histopathological examination of the rectal biopsies of the PI-IBS when compared with controls. There can be at least three scenarios: a prolonged normal inflammatory response, an augmented pathological inflammatory response in these patients, or there is a certain group of patients with particular characteristics that have a higher susceptibility [44, 58–60]. Anyway, there is not yet a firm conclusion.

2.2. Barrier function

The gut barrier function is important in modulating the gut inflammation [26, 61]. The barrier has multiple roles and its integrity is essential for a normal functionality of the digestive system [61]. An impaired barrier could facilitate the passage of inflammatory triggers that might induce changes in the gut. An increased permeability of the barrier might expose various structures to antigen contact [31].

2.3. Cholinergic system

There is another important piece in the complex domino of Inflammation – the so-called "cholinergic anti-inflammatory pathway" [34, 62, 63]. We did not intend to review the data regarding this system as there are multiple reviews [34] that have already analyzed the evidence, but to find the studies that support the interrelation with inflammation in IBS. Dinan et al. [64] investigated several cytokines, such as interleukin (IL): IL-6, IL-8, IL-10, and the growth hormone in the two arms of the study. They found that only IL-6 and the growth hormone in the group of IBS patients were overproduced when compared with controls after the administration of pyridostigmine that might suggest the implication of the cholinergic system [64].

2.4. Low-grade inflammation

More and more data sustain the hypotheses of a low-grade inflammation in IBS [65–67]. The fine line between normal to a pathological inflammatory response is still difficult to set. There is a low-grade inflammation of the gut that has been already acknowledged and literature data supports the putative role of the low-grade inflammation in IBS [65–68]. Several articles addressed this issue, some authors investigated tissue samples [23], while others assessed blood or stool samples [69–72] in order to detect and determine the inflammation status in IBS patients.

There are already numerous studies that assessed erythrocyte sedimentation rate, C-reactive protein (CRP) from blood sample, fecal calprotectin, and/or lactoferin in order to detect their presence in IBS and/or to calculate their predictive values [71–73]. Valuable information was provided by a meta-analysis, although that assessed their cut-off values in order to exclude inflammatory bowel diseases [74].

There are limited data regarding the presence of high-sensibility CRP [69] in IBS, but results indicate that when compared with healthy subjects, levels of high sensibility CRP are statistically significantly higher in IBS patients ($P < 0.001$) [69]. So literature data supports the presence of low-grade inflammation in IBS since the levels of high-sensibility CRP, though were still within the normal range, were higher in IBS than in controls [69].

A similar situation is for calprotectin, which is used mainly for differential diagnosis of inflammatory bowel diseases [73], but there are also studies that showed increased levels of calprotectin in IBS patients when comparing the values of those of healthy controls [72].

In the search to quantify the levels of inflammation, many authors proposed various biomarkers, and others proposed multiple biomarkers such as a panel or a set of markers [75, 76].

2.5. Genes and inflammation in IBS

Genetic factors have also been suspected as being involved in the inflammation in IBS.

Regarding genes and polymorphism, there are several studies that have assessed gene polymorphism, of which IL-10 and α tumor necrosis factor are some of the ones that are being intensively investigated [77–79].

As for the other studies that addressed IBS, their findings are inconsistent since some of the studies that assessed IL-10 genotypes in IBS patients versus controls showed high-producer genotype for IL-10 had a lower frequency statistically significant in IBS than in controls ($P = 0.003$) [79], and other studies did not find statistically significant difference of IL-10 polymorphism in IBS patients [78]. Schmulson et al. [78] assessed two polymorphisms: IL-10 (-1082G/A) and α tumor necrosis factor (-308G/A) in IBS patients and compared them with controls. There were no statistically significant differences between IBS and controls regarding either of the two polymorphisms.

There are also other studies besides these that assessed single nucleotide polymorphisms and more complex studies such as genome-wide association studies [80].

2.6. New hypotheses

There is a growing interest in applying the latest techniques used in molecular biology also for the study of IBS, such as the study of microRNA—miRNAs [81], small interfering RNA—siRNAs [82] or new approaches such as meta-omics [83].

Recently, new directions have been proposed in the study of the etiopathogenesis of IBS [81, 84]. The role of stem cells has been already intensively researched [85, 86], even in inflammatory bowel diseases [87], but these potent cells have raised interest about their role or potential use in IBS.

Very recent data advances the hypotheses that intestinal stem cells might be involved in the inflammatory paths discussed in IBS [84, 88]. Due to their properties, stem cells not only are able to respond to pathogens but also may modulate the spectrum of answers by their secretory functions [84, 89]. These stem cells might also represent therapeutic targets [84], but future studies to identify a specific target, either structural or functional, of the stem cells are mandatory.

The scientific community is eager to develop and improve current technologies, both for identifying new therapeutic targets and also for new treatment.

3. Anti-inflammatory treatment

Treatment of IBS still represents a challenge for clinicians. Due to the marked heterogeneity of the IBS subtypes, we will address anti-inflammatory agents used or those with potential use in IBS. Considering the multifactorial etiology, there are authors who propose a treatment determined by the main pathological path that led to IBS [4]. Literature data are limited concerning pharmacological anti-inflammatory classes studied in IBS as well as for the number of the members of these pharmacological classes that were investigated. Since we cannot still establish the main cause that led to IBS, an etiopathogenetic treatment is not possible, and some are currently being developed; a main aim in the treatment of IBS still is to alleviate the symptoms [1]. Though there are few studies that assessed anti-inflammatory classes or members of these classes in IBS, there is an intensive research activity into unraveling new targets and new treatments [90]. There are ongoing trials [91] and research programs and networks [92] that bring valuable information for a deeper understanding of IBS.

4. Aminosalicylic acid agents

Since the discovery of 5-aminosalicylic acid agents (5-ASA) by Svartz [93] and afterward with their active properties being described by Azad et al. [94], these agents were intensively researched as well as used in clinical practice [95]. The 5-ASA derivates have been used in several inflammatory conditions such as the inflammatory bowel disorders [95]. There are already consistent data regarding the efficacy of 5-ASA in ulcerative colitis [95] as well as regarding their safety. The rationale for prescribing 5-ASA agents in IBS is represented by their anti-inflammatory properties and is the result of several mechanisms [96].

Article	Type of article	Conclusions
Min et al. [97]	Letter	In selected subgroups of IBS might be efficient
Törnblom et al. [98]	Commentaries	In selected subgroups of IBS might be efficient
Lazaraki et al. [99]	Review	Inconclusive regarding the use of mesalasine in IBS
Camilleri et al. [100]	Review	Inconclusive, though some studies show a positive effect on pain, results were not replicated by others
Xue et al. [101]	Letter	Inconclusive—analyzed impact of mesalazine on gut microbiota
Hanevik et al. [102]	Letter + pilot CT	Inefficient
Farup et al. [103]	Letter	Inconclusive – authors underline that Andrews et al. [108] did not analyze drop out patients in their study

Table 1. Articles reviewing the use of 5-ASA in IBS.

Though there are few original studies, there are also reviews that analyze the use of 5-ASA in IBS (**Table 1**). Literature data indicate that in certain group of patients such as those with

http://dx.doi.org/10.5772/66193

PI-IBS, especially the IBS with diarrhoea (IBS-D) subtype could benefit, at least for a certain period of the anti-inflammatory effects of this class (see **Tables 1** and **2**). Regarding the length of treatment, dosing, and schemes of treatment, there are few data in the literature, and there is no study to assess all of this. Future studies are required in order to configure an a priori set of features regarding what type of IBS patient is likely to respond to 5-ASA treatment, as well as the regimen and dosing.

Article	Type of article, type of IBS	Dose and time of treatment	Conclusions
Barbara et al. [104]	Placebo-controlled trial (CT), multicentre IBS	800 mg tid, 12 weeks	Mesalazine treatment was not statistically significant or more efficient than placebo (P = 0.870). In certain groups of patients, it might be useful.
Lam et al. [105]	CT, IBS-D	2 g/day—2 weeks, if tolerated 2 g bid—11 weeks	In certain groups of selected IBS-D patients, it might be efficient, although there is no clear evidence of it being useful.
Bafutto et al. [106]	Pilot study, IBS-D	Various dosing—in the fourth groups	May be useful in certain groups of patients.
Tuteja et al. [107]	CT, PI-IBS	1.6 g bid, 12 weeks	No statistically significant improvement of symptoms ($P \geq 0.11$) nor QOL ($P \geq 0.16$).
Andrews et al. [108]	Pilot study, IBS-D	1.5 g bid, 4 weeks	Significant improvement of pain.
Bafutto et al. [109]	CT, IBS-D	800 mg tid, 30 days	Significant improvement of total symptom score, inclusive of pain. ($P < 0.0001$)
Dorofeyev et al. [110]	CT, IBS, all subtypes	500 mg qid, 28 days	Statistical improvement of abdominal pain ($P < 0.01$) as well as some histopathological aspects.
Hanevik et al. [102]	Letter + pilot CT	800 mg bid, 6 weeks	Inefficient.
Corinaldesi et al. [111]	CT, IBS	800 mg tid, 8 weeks	Mesalazine significantly improved only general well-being ($P = 0.038$), having no significant statistic effect regarding bloating ($P = 0.177$), abdominal pain ($P = 0.084$), or bowel habits.
Preobrazhenskii [112]*	Study	4–6 g daily, not shown	Efficient.

*Articles in other languages (Russian) or full text could not be retrieved.

Table 2. Studies assessing 5-ASA agents in IBS.

4.1. Acetylsalicylic acid

Regarding the use of acetylsalicylic acid, we have identified just one study that assessed it in relation to IBS, but the purpose of the study was to determine if certain anti-inflammatory drugs could induce constipation [113]. In fact, the study assessed that the use of some anti-inflammatory drugs among acetylsalicylic acid was related to constipation. [113].

4.2. Mast cell stabilizers

Mast cell stabilizers (cromoglycate and ketotifen) have been tested in IBS, but there are very few literature data concerning this class of drugs. Also, the criteria used for diagnosing IBS were different; therefore, there is no uniformity when comparing these studies. Subsequent studies are mandatory in order to have the answer: which IBS patients are suited to a mast cell stabilizer treatment and what is the dosing, or what is a suitable regimen.

4.3. Ketotifen

Klooker et al. [114] investigated ketotifen, suggesting that it can reduce visceral hypersensitivity and improve the quality of life. Though there is just one study to investigate ketotifen in IBS patients, there has already been questions about its safety [115]. For certain other studies, to assess this class for IBS treatment is mandatory in order to grade the levels of evidence. Although there is just one study with positive results, we also consider encouraging these results [33], and we strongly feel that there are more therapeutic options that have not yet been explored.

4.4. Cromoglycate

Regarding cromoglycate, there are several studies that assessed it in IBS patients. Literature data suggest that they could have a beneficial role in certain groups of patients, especially in those who have also food allergies or intolerances (see **Table 3**). There are methodological issues concerning these studies; so in order to reduce some of the biases, rigorous parallel studies are needed.

Article	Conclusion
Leri et al. [116]	Efficient (in conjunction with dietary exclusions in IBS patients with food intolerance)
Stefanini et al. [117]	Efficient (in IBS patients with food intolerance)
Grazioli et al. [118]	Efficient (in pediatric IBS patients with food intolerance)
Stefanini et al. [119]	Efficient (in IBS patients with food intolerance)
Lunardi et al. [120]	Efficient (in IBS patients with food intolerance)
Paganelli et al. [121]	Inconclusive
Antico et al. [122]*	–
Stefanini et al. [123]	Efficient
Tomecki et al.* [124]	Inefficient

*Article in other languages than English (Polish, Italian) also could not be retrieved.

Table 3. Articles that assessed cromoglycate in IBS.

4.5. Montelukast

There is just one report of the use of montelukast in IBS stating a positive effect [125]. Considering the pathways that are involved in the pathogenesis of IBS, it seems reasonable that the authors proposed and used it. The wonder is that there are so few data regarding it, though there are data regarding IBS and allergies [29]. Montelukast might be an option for the patients who have IBS and allergic conditions, but there is a lack of studies to address this issue. Rigorous trials with such drugs are needed in order to conclude about their use in IBS.

4.6. Corticosteroids

Some authors even proposed corticosteroids as anti-inflammatory agents in IBS [126]. A short course-3 weeks, 30 mg prednisolone/day was administered to PI-IBS patients and compared with placebo. There was no statistically significant difference between the number of enterochromaffin cells between patients treated with prednisolone and those that received placebo ($P = 0.5$). Though for the reduction of the number of T lymphocytes in the lamina propria. Dunlop et al. [126] found a statistically significant difference that favors prednisolone, there was no improvement regarding several symptoms of IBS.

Due to their known side effects, one study investigated the impact of using oral steroids, showing that they do not have a higher risk for inducing IBS symptoms in adults under 40 years [127].

We conducted a search on PubMed search motor between 1–21st July 2016 using multiple strategies as seen in **Table 4**. There is just one study that assessed the corticoid therapy in IBS, though there are several authors who consider corticosteroids as a reasonable treatment option in certain subgroups of IBS patients (**Table 4**).

Strategy	Results	Appropriate	Inappropriate
"Corticosteroids, irritable bowel syndrome"	91	2 [127, 128]	89
"Corticosteroids, IBS"	64	1 [128]	63
"Prednisone, irritable bowel syndrome"	5	0	5
"Prednisolone, irritable bowel syndrome"	12	1 [126]	11
"Prednisolone, IBS"	5	1 [127]	4
"Budesonide, irritable bowel syndrome"	10	1 [128]	9

Table 4. Results retrieved by several search strategies on PubMed search motor.

4.7. Imunglobulin E antibody (Omalizumab)

There is just one study that addresses this issue [28], which presents a case of a patient that had concurrently IBS and asthma. The patient received an IgE antibody with a major improvement of IBS symptoms. These results suggest that in certain subgroups of patients with concurrent diseases as IBS and atopic status, or extra-intestinal symptoms, IgE antibodies might be useful.

5. Conclusions

Inflammation remains an important pathway involved in the pathogenesis of IBS. Despite the high interest in the field of functional gastrointestinal disorders, till now, researchers have not entirely discovered all the pieces of the complex puzzle that is the etiopathogenesis of IBS, or all of the components of the pathways that finally lead to IBS.

Newer techniques allow detection and promote research of mediators that are involved in inflammation, even in low amounts. Also, the new technologies are able to identify new structures, as well as their potential role to be targeted by pharmacotherapeutic agents.

Results suggest that there are potential pharmacological classes, alongside with potential therapeutic targets that deserve to be reassessed for IBS.

Recent data supports further research of the pathways and structures involved, as well as assessment of not only the newer agents that are currently being developed but also of some of the available ones that do not have sufficient evidence. Emerging therapies that target inflammation are under evaluation, in trials. A multidrug or a multidisciplinary approach needs to be considered in cases that fail to respond to current treatment or to a single therapy, heading toward the current trend, of a personalized medicine.

Abbreviations

5-Aminosalicylic acid agents: 5-ASA

Bis in die: bid

C reactive protein: CRP

Irritable bowel syndrome: IBS

IBS with diarrhoea: IBS-D

Immunoglobulin: Ig

Interleukin: IL

Quarter in die: qid

Quality of life: QOL

Placebo-controlled trial: CT

Postinfectious IBS: PI-IBS

Postdysenteric IBS: PD-IBS

Ter in die: tid

http://dx.doi.org/10.5772/66193

Author details

Alexandra Chira[1], Romeo Ioan Chira[2] and Dan Lucian Dumitrascu[1*]

*Address all correspondence to: ddumitrascu@umfcluj.ro

1 - 2nd Medical Clinic, Department of Internal Medicine, "Iuliu Hatieganu" University of Medicine and Pharmacy Cluj-Napoca, Romania

2 - 1st Medical Clinic, Department of Internal Medicine, Div. Gastroenterology, "Iuliu Hatieganu" University of Medicine and Pharmacy Cluj-Napoca, Romania

References

[1] Drossman DA, Camilleri M, Mayer EA, Whitehead WE. AGA technical review on irritable bowel syndrome. Gastroenterology. 2002;123(6):2108–31.

[2] Bellini M, Gambaccini D, Stasi C, Urbano MT, Marchi S, Usai-Satta P. Irritable bowel syndrome: a disease still searching for pathogenesis, diagnosis and therapy. World J Gastroenterol. 2014;20(27):8807–20.

[3] Barbara G, De Giorgio R, Stanghellini V, Cremon C, Corinaldesi R. A role for inflammation in irritable bowel syndrome? Gut. 2002;51 Suppl 1:i41–4.

[4] Malagelada JR, Malagelada C. Mechanism-oriented therapy of irritable bowel syndrome. Adv Ther. 2016;33(6):877–93.

[5] Chumpitazi BP, Shulman RJ. Underlying molecular and cellular mechanisms in childhood irritable bowel syndrome. Mol Cell Pediatr. 2016;3(1):11.

[6] Mayer EA. Gut feelings: the emerging biology of gut-brain communication. Nat Rev Neurosci. 2011;12(8):453–66.

[7] Jones MP, Dilley JB, Drossman D, Crowell MD. Brain-gut connections in functional GI disorders: anatomic and physiologic relationships. Neurogastroenterol Motil. 2006;18(2):91–103.

[8] James W. What is an emotion? Mind. 1884;9:188–205.

[9] Fichna J, Storr MA. Brain-gut interactions in IBS. Front Pharmacol. 2012;3:127.

[10] Koloski NA, Jones M, Talley NJ. Evidence that independent gut-to-brain and brain-to-gut pathways operate in the irritable bowel syndrome and functional dyspepsia: a 1-year population-based prospective study. Aliment Pharmacol Ther. 2016;44(6):592–600.

[11] Longstreth GF, Thompson WG, Chey WD, Houghton LA, Mearin F, Spiller RC. Functional bowel disorders. Gastroenterology. 2006;130(5):1480–91.

[12] Grover M, Herfarth H, Drossman DA. The functional-organic dichotomy: postinfectious irritable bowel syndrome and inflammatory bowel disease-irritable bowel syndrome. Clin Gastroenterol Hepatol. 2009;7(1):48–53.

[13] Berrill JW, Green JT, Hood K, Campbell AK. Symptoms of irritable bowel syndrome in patients with inflammatory bowel disease: examining the role of sub-clinical inflammation and the impact on clinical assessment of disease activity. Aliment Pharmacol Ther. 2013;38(1):44–51.

[14] Celsus AC. De Medicina, praef. iii. 4.

[15] Rather LJ. Disturbance of function (functio laesa): the legendary fifth cardinal sign of inflammation, added by Galen to the four cardinal signs of Celsus. Bull N Y Acad Med 1971;47:303–322.

[16] Baumann H, Gauldie J. The acute phase response. Immunol Today. 1994;15:74–80.

[17] Sell S, editor. Immunology, Immunopathology, and Immunity. 6th ed. Washington, DC: ASM Press; 2001.

[18] Hiatt RB, Katz L. Mast cells in inflammatory conditions of the gastrointestinal tract. Am J Gastroenterol. 1962;37:541–5.

[19] Shea-Donohue T, Stiltz J, Zhao A, Notari L. Mast cells. Curr Gastroenterol Rep. 2010;12(5):349–57.

[20] Zhang L, Song J, Hou X. Mast cells and irritable bowel syndrome: from the bench to the bedside. J Neurogastroenterol Motil. 2016; 22(2):181–92.

[21] Bischoff SC, Kramer S. Human mast cells, bacteria, and intestinal immunity. Immunol Rev. 2007; 217:329–37.

[22] Barbara G, Stanghellini V, De Giorgio R, Cremon C, Cottrell GS, Santini D, et al. Activated mast cells in proximity to colonic nerves correlate with abdominal pain in irritable bowel syndrome. Gastroenterology. 2004;126(3):693–702.

[23] Chadwick VS, Chen W, Shu D, Paulus B, Bethwaite P, Tie A, et al. Activation of the mucosal immune system in irritable bowel syndrome. Gastroenterology. 2002; 122(7): 1778–83.

[24] O'Sullivan M, Clayton N, Breslin NP, Harman I, Bountra C, McLaren A, et al. Increased mast cells in the irritable bowel syndrome. Neurogastroenterol Motil. 2000;12(5):449–57.

[25] Cremon C, Gargano L, Morselli-Labate AM, Santini D, Cogliandro RF, De Giorgio R, et al. Mucosal immune activation in irritable bowel syndrome: gender-dependence and association with digestive symptoms. Am J Gastroenterol. 2009; 104(2):392–400.

[26] Camilleri M, Lasch K, Zhou W. Irritable bowel syndrome: methods, mechanisms, and pathophysiology. The confluence of increased permeability, inflammation, and pain in

irritable bowel syndrome. Am J Physiol Gastrointest Liver Physiol. 2012; 303(7):G775–85.

[27] Coca A, Cooke R. On the classification of the phenomena of hypersensitiveness. J Immunol; 1923 8: 163–182.

[28] Pearson JS, Niven RM, Meng J, Atarodi S, Whorwell PJ. Immunoglobulin E in irritable bowel syndrome: another target for treatment? A case report and literature review. Therap Adv Gastroenterol. 2015;8(5):270–7.

[29] Vara EJ, Valeur J, Hausken T, Lied GA. Extra-intestinal symptoms in patients with irritable bowel syndrome: related to high total IgE levels and atopic sensitization? Scand J Gastroenterol. 2016;51(8):908–13.

[30] Ohman L, Simren M. Pathogenesis of IBS: role of inflammation, immunity and neuroimmune interactions. Nat Rev Gastroenterol Hepatol. 2010;7(3):163–73.

[31] Spiller RC, Jenkins D, Thornley JP, Hebden JM, Wright T, Skinner M, et al. Increased rectal mucosal enteroendocrine cells, T lymphocytes, and increased gut permeability following acute *Campylobacter enteritis* and in post-dysenteric irritable bowel syndrome. Gut. 2000;47(6):804–11.

[32] Goral V, Kucukoner M, Buyukbayram H. Mast cells count and serum cytokine levels in patients with irritable bowel syndrome. Hepatogastroenterology. 2010;57(101):751–4.

[33] O'Sullivan M. Therapeutic potential of ketotifen in irritable bowel syndrome (IBS) may involve changes in mast cells at sites beyond the rectum. Gut. 2011;60(3):423; author reply.

[34] Pavlov VA, Wang H, Czura CJ, Friedman SG, Tracey KJ. The cholinergic anti-inflammatory pathway: a missing link in neuroimmunomodulation. Mol Med. 2003;9(5-8): 125–34.

[35] Schmulson M, Pulido-London D, Rodriguez O, Morales-Rochlin N, Martinez-Garcia R, Gutierrez-Ruiz MC, et al. Lower serum IL-10 is an independent predictor of IBS among volunteers in Mexico. Am J Gastroenterol. 2012;107(5):747–53.

[36] Bashashati M, Rezaei N, Shafieyoun A, McKernan DP, Chang L, Ohman L, et al. Cytokine imbalance in irritable bowel syndrome: a systematic review and meta-analysis. Neurogastroenterol Motil. 2014;26(7):1036–48.

[37] Macsharry J, O'Mahony L, Fanning A, Bairead E, Sherlock G, Tiesman J, et al. Mucosal cytokine imbalance in irritable bowel syndrome. Scand J Gastroenterol. 2008;43(12): 1467–76.

[38] Watkins LR, Maier SF, Goehler LE. Cytokine-to-brain communication: a review and analysis of alternative mechanisms. Life Sci 57:1011–26. 1995.

[39] Elmquist JK, Scammell TE, Saper CB. Mechanisms of CNS response to systemic immune challenge: the febrile response. Trends Neurosci 20:565–9.

[40] Posserud I, Ersryd A, Simren M. Functional findings in irritable bowel syndrome. World J Gastroenterol. 2006;12(18):2830–8.

[41] Tanaka Y, Kanazawa M, Fukudo S, Drossman DA. Biopsychosocial model of irritable bowel syndrome. J Neurogastroenterol Motil. 2011;17(2):131–9.

[42] Farzaei MH, Bahramsoltani R, Abdollahi M, Rahimi R. The role of visceral hypersensitivity in irritable bowel syndrome: pharmacological targets and novel treatments. J Neurogastroenterol Motil. 2016;22(4):558–574.

[43] Chaudhary NA, Truelove SC. The irritable colon syndrome. A study of the clinical features, predisposing causes, and prognosis in 130 cases. Q J Med. 1962;31:307–22.

[44] Gwee KA, Collins SM, Read NW, Rajnakova A, Deng Y, Graham JC, et al. Increased rectal mucosal expression of interleukin 1beta in recently acquired post-infectious irritable bowel syndrome. Gut. 2003;52(4):523–6.

[45] Rodriguez LA, Ruigomez A. Increased risk of irritable bowel syndrome after bacterial gastroenteritis: cohort study. BMJ. 1999;318(7183):565–6.

[46] Thabane M, Kottachchi DT, Marshall JK. Systematic review and meta-analysis: The incidence and prognosis of post-infectious irritable bowel syndrome. Aliment Pharmacol Ther. 2007;26(4):535–44.

[47] McKendrick MW, Read NW. Irritable bowel syndrome—post salmonella infection. J Infect. 1994;29(1):1–3.

[48] Spiller R, Garsed K. Postinfectious irritable bowel syndrome. Gastroenterology. 2009;136(6):1979–88.

[49] Kim HS, Lim JH, Park H, Lee SI. Increased immunoendocrine cells in intestinal mucosa of postinfectious irritable bowel syndrome patients 3 years after acute Shigella infection—an observation in a small case control study. Yonsei Med J. 2010;51(1):45–51.

[50] Grover M. Role of gut pathogens in development of irritable bowel syndrome. Indian J Med Res. 2014;139(1):11–8.

[51] Okhuysen PC, Jiang ZD, Carlin L, Forbes C, DuPont HL. Post-diarrhea chronic intestinal symptoms and irritable bowel syndrome in North American travelers to Mexico. Am J Gastroenterol. 2004;99(9):1774–8.

[52] Andresen V, Lowe B, Broicher W, Riegel B, Fraedrich K, von Wulffen M, et al. Post-infectious irritable bowel syndrome (PI-IBS) after infection with Shiga-like toxin-producing Escherichia coli (STEC) O104:H4: a cohort study with prospective follow-up. United Eur Gastroenterol J. 2016;4(1):121–31.

[53] Wadhwa A, Al Nahhas MF, Dierkhising RA, Patel R, Kashyap P, Pardi DS, et al. High risk of post-infectious irritable bowel syndrome in patients with Clostridium difficile infection. Aliment Pharmacol Ther. 2016;44(6):576–82.

[54] Marshall JK, Thabane M, Borgaonkar MR, James C. Postinfectious irritable bowel syndrome after a food-borne outbreak of acute gastroenteritis attributed to a viral pathogen. Clin Gastroenterol Hepatol. 2007;5(4):457–60.

[55] Wensaas KA, Langeland N, Hanevik K, Morch K, Eide GE, Rortveit G. Irritable bowel syndrome and chronic fatigue 3 years after acute giardiasis: historic cohort study. Gut. 2012;61(2):214–9.

[56] Azizian M, Basati G, Abangah G, Mahmoudi MR, Mirzaei A. Contribution of Blasto-cystishominis subtypes and associated inflammatory factors in development of irritable bowel syndrome. Parasitol Res. 2016;115(5):2003–9.

[57] Borody TJ, Warren EF, Wettstein A, Robertson G, Recabarren P, Fontella A, et al. Eradication of Dientamoeba fragilis can resolve IBS-like symptoms. J Gastroenterol Hepatol 17(Suppl):A103. 2002.

[58] Wouters MM, Van Wanrooy S, Nguyen A, Dooley J, Aguilera-Lizarraga J, Van Brabant W, et al. Psychological comorbidity increases the risk for postinfectious IBS partly by enhanced susceptibility to develop infectious gastroenteritis. Gut. 2016;65(8):1279–88.

[59] Collins SM, Piche T, Rampal P. The putative role of inflammation in the irritable bowel syndrome. Gut. 2001;49(6):743–5.

[60] Spiller RC. Postinfectious irritable bowel syndrome. Gastroenterology. 2003;124(6): 1662–71.

[61] Martinez C, Gonzalez-Castro A, Vicario M, Santos J. Cellular and molecular basis of intestinal barrier dysfunction in the irritable bowel syndrome. Gut Liver. 2012;6(3):305–15.

[62] Tracey KJ. The inflammatory reflex. Nature 2002;420:853–9..

[63] Blalock JE. Harnessing a neural-immune circuit to control inflammation and shock. J Exp Med 2002;195:F25–8.

[64] Dinan TG, Clarke G, Quigley EM, Scott LV, Shanahan F, Cryan J, et al. Enhanced cholinergic-mediated increase in the pro-inflammatory cytokine IL-6 in irritable bowel syndrome: role of muscarinic receptors. Am J Gastroenterol. 2008;103(10):2570–6.

[65] Akiho H, Ihara E, Nakamura K. Low-grade inflammation plays a pivotal role in gastrointestinal dysfunction in irritable bowel syndrome. World J Gastrointest Patho-physiol. 2010;1(3):97–105.

[66] Lee E, Schiller LR, Fordtran JS. Quantification of colonic lamina propria cells by means of a morphometric point-counting method. Gastroenterology. 1988;94(2):409–18.

[67] Sinagra E, Pompei G, Tomasello G, Cappello F, Morreale GC, Amvrosiadis G, et al. Inflammation in irritable bowel syndrome: myth or new treatment target? World J Gastroenterol. 2016;22(7):2242–55.

[68] Barbara G, Cremon C, Carini G, Bellacosa L, Zecchi L, De Giorgio R, et al. The immune system in irritable bowel syndrome. J Neurogastroenterol Motil. 2011;17(4):349–59.

[69] Hod K, Dickman R, Sperber A, Melamed S, Dekel R, Ron Y, et al. Assessment of high-sensitivity CRP as a marker of micro-inflammation in irritable bowel syndrome. Neurogastroenterol Motil. 2011;23(12):1105–10.

[70] Hod K, Ringel-Kulka T, Martin CF, Maharshak N, Ringel Y. High-sensitive C-reactive protein as a marker for inflammation in irritable bowel syndrome. J Clin Gastroenterol. 2015.

[71] Chang MH, Chou JW, Chen SM, Tsai MC, Sun YS, Lin CC, et al. Faecal calprotectin as a novel biomarker for differentiating between inflammatory bowel disease and irritable bowel syndrome. Mol Med Rep. 2014;10(1):522–6.

[72] David LE, Surdea-Blaga T, Dumitrascu DL. Semiquantitative fecal calprotectin test in postinfectious and non-postinfectious irritable bowel syndrome: cross-sectional study. Sao Paulo Med J. 2014:0.

[73] Otten CM, Kok L, Witteman BJ, Baumgarten R, Kampman E, Moons KG, et al. Diagnostic performance of rapid tests for detection of fecal calprotectin and lactoferrin and their ability to discriminate inflammatory from irritable bowel syndrome. Clin Chem Lab Med. 2008;46(9):1275–80.

[74] Menees SB, Powell C, Kurlander J, Goel A, Chey WD. A meta-analysis of the utility of C-reactive protein, erythrocyte sedimentation rate, fecal calprotectin, and fecal lactoferrin to exclude inflammatory bowel disease in adults with IBS. Am J Gastroenterol. 2015;110(3):444–54.

[75] Lembo AJ, Neri B, Tolley J, Barken D, Carroll S, Pan H. Use of serum biomarkers in a diagnostic test for irritable bowel syndrome. Aliment Pharmacol Ther. 2009;29(8):834–42.

[76] Jones MP, Chey WD, Singh S, Gong H, Shringarpure R, Hoe N, et al. A biomarker panel and psychological morbidity differentiates the irritable bowel syndrome from health and provides novel pathophysiological leads. Aliment Pharmacol Ther. 2014;39(4):426–37.

[77] Olivo-Diaz A, Romero-Valdovinos M, Gudino-Ramirez A, Reyes-Gordillo J, Jimenez-Gonzalez DE, Ramirez-Miranda ME, et al. Findings related to IL-

8 and IL-10 gene polymorphisms in a Mexican patient population with irritable bowel syndrome infected with blastocystis. Parasitol Res. 2012;111(1):487–91.

[78] Schmulson M, Pulido-London D, Rodriguez O, Morales-Rochlin N, Martinez-Garcia R, Gutierrez-Ruiz MC, et al. IL-10 and TNF-alpha polymorphisms in subjects with irritable bowel syndrome in Mexico. Rev Esp Enferm Dig. 2013;105(7):392–9.

[79] Gonsalkorale WM, Perrey C, Pravica V, Whorwell PJ, Hutchinson IV. Interleukin 10 genotypes in irritable bowel syndrome: evidence for an inflammatory component? Gut. 2003;52(1):91–3.

[80] Ek WE, Reznichenko A, Ripke S, Niesler B, Zucchelli M, Rivera NV, et al. Exploring the genetics of irritable bowel syndrome: a GWA study in the general population and replication in multinational case-control cohorts. Gut. 2015;64(11):1774–82.

[81] Zhou Q, Souba WW, Croce CM, Verne GN. MicroRNA-29a regulates intestinal membrane permeability in patients with irritable bowel syndrome. Gut. 2010;59(6):775–84.

[82] Cenac N, Bautzova T, Le Faouder P, Veldhuis NA, Poole DP, Rolland C, et al. Quantification and potential functions of endogenous agonists of transient receptor potential channels in patients with irritable bowel syndrome. Gastroenterology. 2015;149(2):433–44 e7.

[83] Mondot S, Lepage P. The human gut microbiome and its dysfunctions through the meta-omics prism. Ann N Y Acad Sci. 2016;1372(1):9–19.

[84] Ratanasirintrawoot S, Israsena N. Stem cells in the intestine: possible roles in pathogenesis of irritable bowel syndrome. J Neurogastroenterol Motil. 2016;22(3):367–82.

[85] Ozkul Y, Galderisi U. The impact of epigenetics on mesenchymal stem cell biology. J Cell Physiol. 2016;231(11):2393–401.

[86] Wang Q, Ding G, Xu X. Immunomodulatory functions of mesenchymal stem cells and possible mechanisms. Histol Histopathol. 2016;31(9):949–59.

[87] De Francesco F, Romano M, Zarantonello L, Ruffolo C, Neri D, Bassi N, et al. The role of adipose stem cells in inflammatory bowel disease: from biology to novel therapeutic strategies. Cancer Biol Ther. 2016;17(9):889–898.

[88] Roostaee A, Benoit YD, Boudjadi S, Beaulieu JF. Epigenetics in intestinal epithelial cell renewal. J Cell Physiol. 2016;231(11):2361–7.

[89] Owens BM. Inflammation, innate immunity, and the intestinal stromal cell niche: opportunities and challenges. Front Immunol. 2015;6:319.

[90] Corsetti M, Whorwell P. Novel pharmacological therapies for irritable bowel syndrome. Expert Rev Gastroenterol Hepatol. 2016;10(7):807–15.

[91] International Foundation for Functional Gastrointestinal Disorders, Inc. (IFFGD) [Internet]. 1998–2016. Available from: http://www.aboutibs.org/take-part-in-online-studies.html [Accessed: 2016-07-21]

[92] GENIEUR.EU [Internet]. 2012. Available from: https://genieur.eu/ [Accessed: 2016-06-12]

[93] Svartz N. Salazopyrin, a new sulfanilamide preparation: A. Therapeutic results in rheumatic polyarthritis. B. Therapeutic results in ulcerative colitis. C. Toxic manifestations in treatment with sulfanilamide preparation. Acta Med Scand 1942;11:557–590.

[94] Azad Khan AK, Piris J, Truelove SC. An experiment to determine the active therapeutic moiety of sulphasalazine. Lancet. 1977;2(8044):892-5.

[95] Bohm SK, Kruis W. Long-term efficacy and safety of once-daily mesalazine granules for the treatment of active ulcerative colitis. Clin Exp Gastroenterol. 2014;7:369–83.

[96] Desreumaux P. Understanding the mechanism of 5-ASA in treating colonic inflammation. Gastroenterol Hepatol (N Y). 2008;4(5):319–20.

[97] Min T, Ford AC. Efficacy of mesalazine in IBS. Gut. 2016;65(1):187–8.

[98] Törnblom H, Simren M. In search for a disease-modifying treatment in irritable bowel syndrome. Gut. 2016;65(1):2–3.

[99] Lazaraki G, Chatzimavroudis G, Katsinelos P. Recent advances in pharmacological treatment of irritable bowel syndrome. World J. Gastroenterol. 2014;20(27):8867–85.

[100] Camilleri M. Pharmacological agents currently in clinical trials for disorders in neurogastroenterology. J Clin Invest. 2013;123(10):4111–20.

[101] Xue L, Huang Z, Zhou X, Chen W. The possible effects of mesalazine on the intestinal microbiota. Aliment Pharmacol Ther. 2012;36(8):813–4.

[102] Hanevik K, Dizdar V, Langeland N, Eide GE, Hausken T. Tolerability and effect of mesalazine in postinfectious irritable bowel syndrome. Aliment Pharmacol Ther. 2011;34(2):259–60.

[103] Farup PG. Questions about mesalazine and the irritable bowel syndrome. Aliment Pharmacol Ther. 2011;34(8):1036–7; author reply 7–8.

[104] Barbara G, Cremon C, Annese V, Basilisco G, Bazzoli F, Bellini M, et al. Randomised controlled trial of mesalazine in IBS. Gut. 2016;65(1):82–90.

[105] Lam C, Tan W, Leighton M, Hastings M, Lingaya M, Falcone Y, et al. A mechanistic multicentre, parallel group, randomised placebo-controlled trial of mesalazine for the treatment of IBS with diarrhoea (IBS-D). Gut. 2016;65(1):91-9.

[106] Bafutto M, Almeida JR, Leite NV, Costa MB, Oliveira EC, Resende-Filho J. Treatment of diarrhea-predominant irritable bowel syndrome with mesalazine and/or *Saccharomyces boulardii*. Arq Gastroenterol. 2013;50(4):304–9.

[107] Tuteja AK, Fang JC, Al-Suqi M, Stoddard GJ, Hale DC. Double-blind placebo-controlled study of mesalamine in post-infective irritable bowel syndrome—a pilot study. Scand J Gastroenterol. 2012;47(10):1159–64.

[108] Andrews CN, Griffiths TA, Kaufman J, Vergnolle N, Surette MG, Rioux KP. Mesalazine (5-aminosalicylic acid) alters faecal bacterial profiles, but not mucosal proteolytic activity in diarrhoea-predominant irritable bowel syndrome. Aliment Pharmacol Ther. 2011;34(3):374–83.

[109] Bafutto M, Almeida JR, Leite NV, Oliveira EC, Gabriel-Neto S, Rezende-Filho J. Treatment of postinfectious irritable bowel syndrome and noninfective irritable bowel syndrome with mesalazine. Arq Gastroenterol. 2011;48(1):36–40.

[110] Dorofeyev AE, Kiriyan EA, Vasilenko IV, Rassokhina OA, Elin AF. Clinical, endoscopical and morphological efficacy of mesalazine in patients with irritable bowel syndrome. Clin Exp Gastroenterol. 2011;4:141–53.

[111] Corinaldesi R, Stanghellini V, Cremon C, Gargano L, Cogliandro RF, De Giorgio R, et al. Effect of mesalazine on mucosal immune biomarkers in irritable bowel syndrome: a randomized controlled proof-of-concept study. Aliment Pharmacol Ther. 2009;30(3):245–52.

[112] Preobrazhenskii VN. Salozinal in the treatment of the irritable bowel syndrome in young persons. Ter Arkh. 1999;71(2):37–9.

[113] Chang JY, Locke GR, Schleck CD, Zinsmeister AR, Talley NJ. Risk factors for chronic constipation and a possible role of analgesics. Neurogastroenterol Motil. 2007;19(11):905-11.

[114] Klooker TK, Braak B, Koopman KE, Welting O, Wouters MM, van der Heide S, et al. The mast cell stabiliser ketotifen decreases visceral hypersensitivity and improves intestinal symptoms in patients with irritable bowel syndrome. Gut. 2010;59(9):1213–21.

[115] Reisinger KW, de Haan JJ, Schreinemacher MH. Word of caution before implementing ketotifen for gastrointestinal transit improvement. World J. Gastroenterol. 2013;19(27):4445–6.

[116] Leri O, Tubili S, De Rosa FG, Addessi MA, Scopelliti G, Lucenti W, et al. Management of diarrhoeic type of irritable bowel syndrome with exclusion diet and disodium cromoglycate. Inflammopharmacology. 1997;5(2):153–8.

[117] Stefanini GF, Saggioro A, Alvisi V, Angelini G, Capurso L, di Lorenzo G, et al. Oral cromolyn sodium in comparison with elimination diet in

the irritable bowel syndrome, diarrheic type. Multicenter study of 428 patients. Scand J Gastroenterol. 1995;30(6):535–41.

[118] Grazioli I, Melzi G, Balsamo V, Castellucci G, Castro M, Catassi C, et al. Food intolerance and irritable bowel syndrome of childhood: clinical efficacy of oral sodium cromoglycate and elimination diet. Minerva Pediatr. 1993;45(6):253–8.

[119] Stefanini GF, Prati E, Albini MC, Piccinini G, Capelli S, Castelli E, et al. Oral disodium cromoglycate treatment on irritable bowel syndrome: an open study on 101 subjects with diarrheic type. Am J Gastroenterol. 1992;87(1):55–7.

[120] Lunardi C, Bambara LM, Biasi D, Cortina P, Peroli P, Nicolis F, et al. Double-blind crossover trial of oral sodium cromoglycate in patients with irritable bowel syndrome due to food intolerance. Clin Exp Allergy. 1991;21(5):569–72.

[121] Paganelli R, Fagiolo U, Cancian M, Sturniolo GC, Scala E, D'Offizi GP. Intestinal permeability in irritable bowel syndrome. Effect of diet and sodium cromoglycate administration. Ann Allergy. 1990;64(4):377–80.

[122] Antico A, Soana R, Clivio L, Baioni R. Irritable colon syndrome in intolerance to food additives. Minerva Dietol Gastroenterol. 1989;35(4):219–24.

[123] Stefanini GF, Bazzocchi G, Prati E, Lanfranchi GA, Gasbarrini G. Efficacy of oral disodium cromoglycate in patients with irritable bowel syndrome and positive skin prick tests to foods. Lancet. 1986;1(8474):207–8.

[124] Tomecki R. Ineffectiveness of disodium cromoglycate in the treatment of a diarrheal form of irritable bowel syndrome. Pol Tyg Lek. 1985;40(7):181–2.

[125] Fee WH. Irritable bowel syndrome helped by montelukast. Chest. 2002;122(4):1497.

[126] Dunlop SP, Jenkins D, Neal KR, Naesdal J, Borgaonker M, Collins SM, et al. Randomized, double-blind, placebo-controlled trial of prednisolone in post-infectious irritable bowel syndrome. Aliment Pharmacol Ther. 2003;18(1):77–84.

[127] Huerta C, Garcia Rodriguez LA, Wallander MA, Johansson S. Users of oral steroids are at a reduced risk of developing irritable bowel syndrome. Pharmacoepidemiol Drug Saf. 2003;12(7):583–8.

[128] Crentsil V. Will corticosteroids and other anti-inflammatory agents be effective for diarrhea-predominant irritable bowel syndrome? Med Hypotheses. 2005;65(1):97–102.

Chapter 4

Dietary Management in IBS Patients

Francesca Pasqui, Carolina Poli,
Caterina Magrino and Davide Festi

Additional information is available at the end of the chapter

http://dx.doi.org/10.5772/66192

Abstract

Irritable bowel syndrome (IBS) is a chronic, relapsing functional disorder of the gastrointestinal tract characterized by abdominal pain, bloating, and changes in bowel habits lacking a known structural or anatomic explanation. According to the Rome IV criteria, IBS consists of a set of altered bowel habits over a period of time and includes abdominal pain and discomfort. The pathogenesis of IBS is not completely understood, although it has been noted that various mechanisms are involved determining the onset of symptoms. The risk factors include antibiotics, enteric infection, food intolerance, altered pain perception, altered brain-gut interaction, dysbiosis, increased intestinal permeability, visceral hypersensitivity, and increased activation of the gut mucosal immune system. There has been interest regarding the possible role of food in IBS. Diet is crucial for managing IBS; it plays an important role both in the genesis and in the improvement of symptoms. The aim of the study was to summarize the evidence from the literature, which explains those causes tending to promoting IBS symptoms, such as food content short-chain carbohydrates and the presence of food allergy or food intolerance.

Keywords: IBS, FODMAPs, microbiota, diet, food allergy

1. Introduction

Irritable bowel syndrome (IBS) is a chronic functional gastrointestinal disorder; it is not associated with organic causes which can be detected using current diagnostic tools [1–3]. It is characterized by abdominal pain, distension, bloating and stool irregularities and its prevalence is 10–20%. The prevalence of IBS differs among countries; this may be due to varying application of the diagnostic criteria, demographic differences and other factors, such as lifestyle including physical activity, dietary habits, distress, and pharmacological treatment [4].

The incidence of IBS in women is twofold that of men, the majority in the <50-year-old age group and having a lower socioeconomic status [5]. Symptom severity varies in different patients, from tolerable to severe, possibly interfering with daily activity [6]; in fact, patients with IBS have a reduction in the quality of life and work productivity, and they sometimes tend to isolate themselves socially [5, 7]. Many patients report avoiding social events due to embarrassment from postprandial symptoms and lack of access to toilet facilities [2, 8].

The pathogenesis of IBS is not completely understood, although it has been suggested that various mechanisms are involved [9], such as the use of antibiotics, enteric infection, food intolerance, altered pain perception, altered brain-gut interaction, dysbiosis, increased intestinal permeability, visceral hypersensitivity, and increased activation of the gut mucosal immune system [7].

Since the etiology of IBS is unknown, there is no specific therapeutic strategy; in fact, treatment is often symptomatic, namely the alleviation of symptoms. The diagnosis of IBS is clinical, based on symptoms according to the Rome IV Criteria [10], which have updated the previous criteria:

The term "discomfort" has been eliminated since it was ambiguous for the patients.

In the past, the relative frequency of abdominal pain as a diagnostic criterion had to be at least 3 days a month.

"Improvement of symptoms with defecation" is no longer quoted; instead "related to defecation" is used since a large number of patients did not have improvement in abdominal pain with defecation but, rather, a worsening [3].

Symptom onset should occur at least 6 months before diagnosis, and the symptoms should be present for three successive months [10, 11].

The following IBS subtypes can be identified according to the predominant change in bowel habit:

- (IBS-C) with predominant constipation
- (IBS-D) with diarrhea
- (IBS-M) mixed
- (IBS-U) unsubtyped [1]

Over time, patients may migrate between the different IBS subtypes, most commonly from IBS-C or IBS-D to IBS-M [7].

2. Diet and lifestyle in IBS

As has already been pointed out, IBS patients frequently report that symptom exacerbation occurs after the ingestion of some foods. In fact, it has been reported that approximately 90% of patients voluntarily restrict their diet in order to prevent or improve their symptoms [2, 7]. Over time, excessive limitation of the quality and/or quantity of foods assumed can lead to malnutrition [12, 13].

Furthermore, the occurrence of exaggerated symptoms after food ingestion, such as gastric hypersensitivity to distension, small intestinal hypersensitivity to fat, and hypersensitivity to the effect of gut hormones, acid, capsaicin, and the products of colonic fermentation, has been observed [1, 14, 15].

This exaggerated response to the ingestion of lipids probably reflects the complexity of digestion and absorption, which is also present in physiological conditions. Another aspect regards the short-chain carbohydrates, which are poorly absorbed in the small bowel; therefore, the increased osmotic load increases the intestinal water content.

Short-chain carbohydrate malabsorption leads to their rapid fermentation which, in turn, leads to the production of short-chain fatty acids and gas, mainly hydrogen, carbon dioxide and methane, which may induce the bloating responsible for the abdominal pain [16, 17].

Owing to the strict relationship between food and symptom development present in patients with IBS, therapeutic management includes dietary and lifestyle advice and, in case of necessity, psychotherapy and pharmacological therapy targeted toward the symptoms [18].

In clinical practice, the following items need to be evaluated in patients with IBS, in order to identify their possible pathogenetic role:

1. Fermentable Oligo-, Di-, Monosaccharide and Polyols (FODMAPs)

2. Food allergy

3. Non-celiac gluten sensitivity (NCGS)

4. Interaction between diet and gut microbiota

2.1. FODMAPs

The term FODMAP was first coined by researchers at Monash University in Melbourne, Australia, to describe a group of short-chain carbohydrates and polyols [16, 19].

In recent years, the intake of FODMAPs has increased in Western diets, in particular, that of fructose due to the greater availability and consumption of fruit and fruit juice, and the extensive use of high fructose corn syrup in a wide variety of processed food and beverages [20].

2.1.1. Fructose

Fructose is a monosaccharide which is dose-dependently and variably absorbed; when an excess of glucose is present, it is taken up by a low-capacity facultative transporter called GLUT 5 [16, 21].

When the concentration of fructose is greater in the lumen with respect to that in the epithelial cells, a gradient of concentration is created which permits the fructose, by means of transport proteins, to enter into the interior of the epithelial cells, thereby being absorbed.

The transport proteins, however, saturate at low fructose concentrations which, in turn, lead to malabsorption [22]. However, when fructose is present with glucose, the fructose is taken up more efficiently by means of the GLUT2 transporter. The fructose-glucose ratio is crucial for adequate fructose absorption, and a 1:1 ratio is considered optimal [16, 21]. It has been observed that 40% of the population has "fructose malabsorption" due to its scarce capacity of absorption at the intestinal level [22–24].

2.1.2. Fructans and galacto-oligosaccharides (GOS)

Fructans are oligo or polysaccharides made up of small chains of fructose units having a terminal molecule of glucose. Fructans with a 2–9 unit length are defined as oligofructose and those with >10 units as inulins [22, 25, 26]. Due to the lack of enzymes capable of completely hydrolyzing the glycosidic bonds of these polysaccharides, the human body absorbs only 5–15% of the fructans; the fructans which are not absorbed are released into the colon where they undergo fermentation [26]. Wheat represents the major source of fructans in the diet (1–4%) [22, 27]. Rye also contains fructans; its chain length is longer than that found in wheat, which could make it less osmotically active or less rapidly fermented. The principal sources of galacto-oligosaccharides (GOS) are raffinose, which is made up of one fructose, one glucose, and one galactose molecule, and stachyose, which has the same composition as raffinose with the exception of having an additional galactose molecule. The human body is not capable of digesting raffinose and stachyose due to the lack of enzymes able to hydrolyze the bonds. Galactooligosaccharides are present, above all, in vegetables [22, 28]. Fructans and galactooligosaccharides are defined as "prebiotics" due to their ability to selectively stimulate the growth of beneficial colonic bacteria, specifically *Bifidobacteria* and *Lactobacilli* [16, 29, 30].

2.1.3. Polyols

Sorbitol, mannitol, xylitol, maltitol, erythirol, polydextrose, and isomalt are sugar alcohols. Sorbitol and mannitol are the major types found in food, and they are found naturally in fruits and vegetables, or as added sweeteners in low-calorie food products [16]. They are identified on food packaging with the following numbers: E420 (sorbitol), E421 (mannitol), E965 (maltitol), E967 (xylitol), and E953 (isomalt) [22]. Their rates of absorption depend largely on molecular size; their absorption is passive and varies between individuals [22, 31].

2.1.4. Lactose

Lactose is a disaccharide consisting of galactose bound to glucose; intestinal absorption requires hydrolysis to its component monosaccharides by brush-border enzyme lactase. Lactase begins its activity at approximately the eighth week of gestation; activity increases until week 34 and the peak of activity is at birth [32].

After the first few months of life, lactase activity begins to decrease; this condition is defined as "lactase non-persistence." However, approximately 30% of the population retains its capacity to digest lactose (lactase persistence); in particular, this is observed in the populations of Northern Europe as a result of the introduction of dairy farming approximately 10,000 years ago [17, 33]. Only 50% of lactase activity is necessary for the efficient digestion of lactose without causing symptoms of intolerance [17]. Lactase deficiency determines lactose intolerance and is defined as markedly reduced brush-border lactase activity, whereas lactose malabsorption occurs when a substantial amount of lactose is not absorbed in the intestine. Three distinct forms of deficiency exist: congenital, primary and secondary. The congenital form is extremely rare; it can be observed in newborns and is characterized by diarrhea from the first exposure to breast milk and by growth defects [32]. "Primary lactase deficiency" refers to the condition of lactase non-persistence, already described above, whereas secondary or acquired lactase deficiency refers to the loss of lactase activity in individuals with lactase persistence. This could be secondary to a gastrointestinal disease, which damages the brush border and is usually reversible. The primary aim in treating lactose intolerance is the improvement of symptoms. Therefore, it is necessary to reduce the malabsorption, and limiting the intake of the lactose found in milk and its derivatives is recommended.

In order to avoid the onset of symptoms, patients with self-reported lactose intolerance, even those with IBS, can ingest at least 12 g of lactose per day [17, 34, 35]. However, it has also been observed that, in many individuals, the restriction of lactose alone was not sufficient for improving functional GI symptoms. This is because lactose intolerance is part of a wider intolerance to FODMAPs [17, 36]. Lactase enzyme replacement products can be found commercially, but they should be used only by those individuals who have isolated lactose intolerance and wish to enjoy dairy products [17]. It is important to remember that dairy products are the major source of calcium in many individuals; therefore, it is reasonable to recommend increasing calcium intake from other foods, water rich in calcium or supplements, especially in the presence of other risk factors for osteoporosis [17].

2.2. Food allergy

Food allergy is an adverse immune response toward food proteins or a form of food intolerance associated with a hypersensitive immune response. There are three types of food allergies: IgE mediated, mixed IgE/non-IgE, which involves eosinophilic and other cellular components, and non-IgE mediated [37].

Food allergy has rapidly increased in prevalence. It suggests the important role of environmental factors in disease susceptibility [37]. Of the 20–30% of the population reported to be allergic or to have allergic children, the presence of allergy can be ascertained in only 6–8% of children under 5 years of age and in 3–4% of adults [38, 39].

In the presence of food allergies, a small quantity of food can cause an immediate reaction. The symptoms involving the gastrointestinal tract can include nausea, vomiting, abdominal cramps and diarrhea, other signs can involve the oropharyngeal tract or the skin [38, 40]. There has been interest regarding the possible role of food allergies in IBS, but few data are available to support this association [38].

In order to exclude food allergies, it is necessary to proceed on the basis of the results of the following tests:

1. *Total serum IgE*: High values may indicate the presence of some food allergies [38, 41].
2. *Immunoglobulin G (IgG):* It often produces false positive, and it is not recommended, as a diagnostic test, by national and international guidelines [38, 42].
3. *The radioallergosorbent test (RAST) of food/serum food-specific IgE:* A direct correlation exists between increasing concentrations of food-specific serum IgE and the probability that an individual will react to an ingested food [38, 43–45].
4. *The skin prick or scratch test:* Positivity indicates the presence of IgE to specific foods [38, 42, 44–47].

Furthermore, it is necessary to make an interview and administer an accurate food questionnaire in order to identify the correlation between specific food and symptoms.

2.3. Non-celiac gluten sensitivity (NCGS)

Currently, the gluten-related disorders actually documented are celiac disease (CD), non-celiac gluten sensitivity (NCGS) and wheat allergy (WA) [48]. Celiac disease is an autoimmune condition, which is characterized by an immunological response to ingesting gluten, which results in small-intestine villous atrophy with increased permeability and malabsorption of nutrients [48, 49].

Wheat allergy is characterized by an IgE-mediated response against various wheat components, which cause gastrointestinal and respiratory symptoms [48–50].

A food allergy to wheat begins with different symptoms as vomiting, abdominal pain, asthma, allergic rhinitis, urticaria/angioedema, acute exacerbation of atopic dermatitis, and exercise-induced anaphylaxis. The prevalence of IgE-mediated food allergies to wheat, confirmed by a food induce, is unknown.

At the moment, the management of IgE-mediated wheat allergy is mainly based on the avoidance of both food and inhaled wheat allergens. Patients allergic to wheat must be trained to identify relevant food allergens on labels, and written instructions should be given to effectively eliminate wheat from their diet [51].

Non-celiac gluten sensitivity is an emerging clinical problem characterized by various manifestations, in particular by IBS-like gastrointestinal symptoms and extra-intestinal symptoms, such as malaise, fatigue, headache, mental confusion, anxiety, sleep abnormality, and skin rash related to the ingestion of gluten-containing foods in patients who are not affected by either celiac disease or wheat allergy [52].

The symptoms generally improve after the removal of wheat products from the diet. Due to the lack of biomarkers, the diagnosis of NCGS is mainly based on clinical criteria [52, 53] after having excluded the presence of CD, WA, gluten ataxia, and dermatitis herpetiformis [52].

Similar to IBS, NCGS affects more young women (in their third decade of life; female:male = 3:1) [52]. The consumption of wheat has increased and is correlated not only to its adaptability and potential for high yields but also to its viscoelasticity, which allows it to be processed into several food items, such as bread, baked products, and pastas [54].

There are two components of wheat which could evoke IBS symptoms: proteins (primarily gluten) and short-chain carbohydrates (primarily fructans and galactans) [52].

Various studies have been carried out to verify which of these two components is responsible for the onset of symptoms. A study was carried out on patients with IBS who autonomously started a gluten-free diet; it was observed that the gastrointestinal symptoms significantly and consistently improved with a low-FODMAP diet, and symptoms did not worsen with either a low- or a high-dose challenge with gluten [54, 55].

Another study involving adults who believed that they had NCGS concluded that it was not gluten to induce the clinical picture [54]. Trials carried out on patients with suspected NCGS support the data regarding a greater improvement of the symptoms with a low-FODMAP diet as compared to a gluten-free diet [56–58].

A recent systematic review regarding NCGS concluded that there is insufficient evidence to support the efficacy of a gluten-free diet for NCGS [59].

2.4. Interaction between diet and microbiota

From birth, the gut microbiota plays various roles in the gastrointestinal tract. Postnatal gut function and immune development are largely influenced by intestinal microbiota. In fact, it has a role in gastrointestinal motility and the immune system, it provides protection against infection, it contributes to the development of gut function and the regulation and maintenance of the intestinal barrier, and it promotes food tolerance. Microbial species promote symbiotic host-bacteria interactions, which are fundamental for human health [12, 60, 61].

The gastrointestinal microbiota is determined by host genetic and environmental factors [12, 60, 62]. The composition of the microbiota varies according to prenatal events, delivery methods, infant feeding, infant care environment, and antibiotic use. Emerging evidence has shown that early microbiota colonization may influence the occurrence of eventual diseases [61]. Gut microbiota interferes with the intestinal functions it can be the cause of irregularity of intestinal sensitivity, motility, neuroimmune signaling, such as the alterations of the mucosal barrier and pattern recognition receptor expression and dysfunctions of the hypothalamus-pituitary-adrenal axis [63].

It has an important role in the digestion of dietary components, resulting in metabolites which may directly or indirectly contribute to IBS symptoms [12]. The vast majority of microbial commensal species give rise to symbiotic host-bacterial interactions, which are fundamental for human health [64]. Disruption and/or imbalance of the establishment of stable normal gut microbiota, dysbiosis, may be associated with the pathogenesis of several gastrointestinal conditions, such as inflammatory bowel disease (IBD) and irritable bowel syndrome, and wider systemic manifestations of disease, such as obesity, type 2 diabetes and atopy [12, 64, 65]. In the healthy gut, intestinal microbiota can prevent the adherence of pathogenic bacteria to the wall of the gastrointestinal tract [66]. In addition, dysbiosis in the gut may facilitate the adhesion of enteric pathogens, which could be associated with IBS symptoms [67]. Alteration of the composition of the normal microbiota and disturbed colonic fermentation in IBS patients may play an important role in the development of IBS symptoms, with a significant increase in the ratio of Firmicutes to Bacteroidetes [65, 68]. Dysregulated intestinal immune function, chronic low-grade mucosal inflammation and increased mucosal permeability and barrier dysfunction have all been suggested to be pathogenic mechanisms in IBS in which the intestinal microbiota might have a role [12, 69, 70]. Part of the etiology of IBS may involve the use of antibiotics; in these cases, probiotics are effective in ameliorating symptoms, even if the consistency of benefits across clinical studies is difficult to discern due to variation in strains, product dosages and the duration of the trials [68, 71–73].

Manipulation of the gut microbiota represents a new strategy for the treatment of IBS. Modulating the gut bacterial composition, expanding the bacterial species considered to be beneficial (*Lactobacilli* and *Bifidobacteria*) and reducing the bacterial species considered to be harmful (*Clostridium, Escherichia coli, Salmonella, Shigella,* and *Pseudomonas*) should attenuate IBS symptoms [63].

Several studies using culture-based and culture-independent methods have shown that the microbiota differs between IBS patients and healthy controls [12, 74, 75].

However, the association between IBS symptoms and specific bacterial species is uncertain [12, 76]. Decreased levels of *Lactobacilli* and *Bifidobacteria,* increased levels of anaerobic bacteria, such as *Streptococci* and *Escherichia coli,* as well as increased ratios of Firmicutes, Bacteroidetes, and *Clostridium* species, have been confirmed in several studies [12, 77, 78]. Studies have indicated that the microbiota, its function and its metabolic output are influenced by dietary patterns [79].

Habitual long-term dietary patterns have been directly linked to intestinal microbial enterotypes. Protein and animal fat intake have been associated with the Bacteroides enterotype, whereas a high-carbohydrate intake has been associated with the Prevotella enterotype [12, 80].

Preliminary data suggest that a diet with a low content of FODMAPs can reduce the growth of important species, such as Bifidobatteri [81]. The effect of short-term dietary interventions on the microbiota composition appears to have only a modest effect [12, 80, 82]. Diet and composition of the microbiota are two major interrelated factors, which can modify susceptibility to food allergy [37].

http://dx.doi.org/10.5772/66192

The number of publications describing an altered microbiota in allergic disease has significantly increased in recent years. The increasing use of antibiotics, in both humans and agriculture, and the increasing consumption of a high-fat/low-fiber diet have had a major impact on the gut microbiota and have been associated with an increased allergic response to food in industrialized countries in recent decades [83–85].

The use of probiotics to stabilize microbial homeostasis seems to be promising, but, to better understand the potential beneficial impact from probiotics, prebiotics, and bacterial-produced metabolites in the treatment of allergic disease, additional studies are needed [85].

3. Role of diet

Therefore, diet is crucial for managing IBS despite the lack of solid evidence involving many dietary recommendations for IBS; this issue must be addressed in clinical practice. The British Dietetic Association and NICE guidelines (National Institute for Health and Clinical Excellence) recommend that dietary and lifestyle advice should be routinely provided to patients [2]:

- Patients with IBS should be educated about the importance of self-help in effectively managing their IBS through information regarding lifestyle, physical activity, diet, and symptom-targeted medication.
- Professionals should encourage people with IBS to use their available leisure time to make relax.
- People should be motivated to increase their activity levels.
- In people with IBS diet and nutrition have to be assessed and general advice should be given:
  - Have regular meals during the day and take time to eat with calm.
  - Avoid skip meals and stay for long time without eating.
  - Drink at least 1500 ml of liquid/day, preferring water or other non-caffeinated drinks.
  - No more than three cups per day of tea and coffee.
  - Reduce alcohol and fizzy drinks.
  - Limit the intake of high-fiber food; reduce the intake of "resistant starch" (RS) because they resist to digestion in the small intestine and reaches the colon intact.
  - No more than three portions of fresh fruit per day.
  - In case of diarrhea, it is advisable to avoid sorbitol, an artificial sweetener found in sugar-free sweets, light drinks, and in some diabetic and diet products.
  - In case of wind and bloating, it is advisable to eat oats and linseeds.
- Healthcare professionals should review the fiber intake of people with IBS, adjusting it while monitoring its effect on the symptoms. People with IBS should be discouraged from eating

insoluble fiber. If an increase in dietary fiber is advised, it should be soluble fiber. People with IBS could try probiotics, and they should take the product for at least 4 weeks while monitoring the effect. Probiotics should be taken at the dosage recommended by the manufacturer.

- Discourage the use of aloe vera in the treatment of IBS.
- If a person's IBS symptoms persist while following general lifestyle and dietary advice, offer advice on additional dietary management.
    - Include single food avoidance and exclusion diets such as a low-FODMAP diet.
    - Only be given by a healthcare professional with expertise in dietary management.

A low-FODMAP diet provides for the restriction of all short-chain carbohydrates by finding low-FODMAP alternatives in each food group. The aim is that of reducing the malabsorption induced by these nutrients and the consequences, such as luminal distension and fermentation caused by the bacteria of the colon, which give rise to the symptoms [52].

In healthy adults, FODMAPs do not cause gastrointestinal symptoms; conversely, in IBS patients, this probably is a consequence of the previously mentioned abnormalities in gut physiology and visceral sensation [7, 86, 87].

There is evidence of low-FODMAP diet efficacy; in fact, it has been observed that it reduces and controls the GI symptoms with respect to a high-FODMAP diet [2, 88, 89], and this has also been confirmed by clinical trials [5, 90].

The low-FODMAP diet was compared with the indications of the NICE guidelines in order to verify which of the two approaches was better in controlling the symptoms.

In particular, in one study, it emerged that there was significantly greater satisfaction with symptom response with the low-FODMAP diet (76%) as compared to the NICE guidelines (54%) [5, 89].

Instead, a recent single-blinded random controlled trial (RCT) compared the efficacy of a low-FODMAP diet to the NICE guidelines for a 4-week period at the end of which an improvement in the IBS Symptom Severity Score (IBS SSS) was observed in both groups but without significant differences. At the end of the study, 56% of the patients on the low FODMAP diet and 46% on the traditional IBS diet responded to the treatment, and the IBS SSS was reduced to ≥ 50 relative to baseline. Food diaries demonstrated good adherence to the dietary advice [16, 91].

A recent meta-analysis, which compared IBS patients who followed a Westernized diet with patient who followed a low FODMAPs diet, showed that adherence to a low-FODMAP diet help to ameliorate all the functional IBS's symptoms and their severity also improving the quality of life score [20].

The symptom with the least improvement was constipation; in fact, a typical FODMAP diet can often be lacking in fiber content. If one decides to follow a low-FODMAP diet, it should

http://dx.doi.org/10.5772/66192

be followed for at least 2–6 weeks in order to be able to verify whether there is effectively an improvement in the symptomology [5].

If patients report improvement, dietary rechallenge with FODMAPs may be tried gradually, that is, one food at a time can be reinserted, starting with small quantities [5]. The risk of inserting more than one food at a time is that of not being able to verify which, effectively, is that responsible for the worsening of the symptoms [5].

Decisions related to the food allowed or to that which should be avoided should always be based on individual tolerance; one valid evaluation instrument is a food diary in which patients have to report what they eat qualitatively, thereby being able to identify potential trigger foods [5].

The effect of a long-term FODMAP diet is not clear; few data are available regarding its long-term efficacy and safety. Presumably, a long-term low-FODMAP diet could lead to nutritional inadequacy. In one study evaluating the effect of fermentable carbohydrate restriction as compared with a control diet, no difference was found in micronutrient intake, except for a lower calcium intake, presumably as a result of the lower intake of dairy products [16, 90].

This might pose a problem principally for children and postmenopausal women [16]. The psychosocial risks of imposing a dietary change and the various difficulties encountered by an IBS patient, difficulties in socialization and eating disorders, such as orthorexia nervosa, should not be underestimated [52, 92].

4. Conclusions

The symptoms of IBS can be similar to those of other pathological conditions; it is necessary to exclude them by means of diagnostic examinations. From a nutritional point of view, the symptoms of IBS patients linked to food as well as to their present food habits must be evaluated carefully in order to reach a nutritional diagnosis and the specific objectives to reach, verifying the relative changes by means of successive checkups. Furthermore, a careful evaluation of the nutritional state is recommended with the aim of identifying, if present, the eventual lack of macro/micronutrients. It is possible to consider a dietetic regimen, which has a behavioral checkup linked to the indications of the NICE guidelines; successively, or in association with the execution of the guidelines, a low-FODMAP diet can be proposed which foresees a reduction in the intake of foods containing high quantities of short-chain carbohydrates and polyols in favor of substitutes for each food group in order to avoid undesired weight losses and nutritional deficits. A low-FODMAP diet must be limited to a precise period of time, and the patient must be monitored by keeping a daily food diary where the food consumed over a 24-h period, the subdivision of the meals and the clinical picture present is reported. Use of a diary makes patients feel more understood, with a consequent perception of greater interest in their problems and needs. With the reduction or disappearance of the clinical picture, the foods previously excluded can be reinserted, one at a time, evaluating individual tolerance with the aim of restoring a complete and balanced diet, always with the help of a food diary.

Author details

Francesca Pasqui*, Carolina Poli, Caterina Magrino and Davide Festi

*Address all correspondence to: francesca.pasqui@unibo.it

Department of Medical and Surgical Sciences, University of Bologna, Bologna, Italy

References

[1] Enck P., Aziz Q., Barbara G., Farmer AD., Fukudo S., Mayer EA., et al. Irritable bowel syndrome. Nat Rev Dis Primer. 2016;2:16014. doi: 10.1038/nrdp.2016.14

[2] Hayes PA., Fraher MH., Quigley EMM. Irritable bowel syndrome: the role of food in pathogenesis and management. Gastroenterol Hepatol. 2014;10:164–74.

[3] Mearin F., Lacy BE., Chang L., Chey WD., Lembo AJ., Simren M., Spiller R. Bowel disorders. Gastroenterology. 2016;150:1393–407. doi: 10.1053/j.gastro.2016.02.031

[4] Nanayakkara WS., Skidmore PM., O'Brien L., Wilkinson TJ., Gearry RB. Efficacy of the low FODMAP diet for treating irritable bowel syndrome: the evidence to date. Clin Exp Gastroenterol. 2016;9:131–42. doi: 10.2147/CEG.S86798

[5] Khan MA., Nusrat S., Khan MI., Nawras A., Bielefeldt K. Low-FODMAP Diet for irritable bowel syndrome: is it ready for prime time? Dig Dis Sci. 2015;60:1169–77. doi: 10.1007/s10620-014-3436-4

[6] Mansueto P., D'Alcamo A., Seidita A., Carroccio A. Food allergy in irritable bowel syndrome: the case of non-celiac wheat sensitivity. World J Gastroenterol. 2015;21:7089–109. doi: 10.3748/wjg.v21.i23.7089

[7] Chey WD., Kurlander J., Eswaran S. Irritable bowel syndrome: a clinical review. JAMA. 2015;313:949. doi: 10.1001/jama.2015.0954

[8] Bertram S., Kurland M., Lydick E., Locke GR., Yawn BP. The patient's perspective of irritable bowel syndrome. J Fam Pract. 2001;50:521–5.

[9] Soares RL. Irritable bowel syndrome: a clinical review. World J Gastroenterol. 2014;20(34):12144–60. doi: 10.3748/wjg.v20.i34.12144

[10] Mearin F., Ciriza C., Mínguez M., Rey E., Mascort JJ., Peña E., Cañones P., Júdez J. Clinical practice guideline: irritable bowel syndrome with constipation and functional constipation in the adult. Rev Esp Enfermedades Dig. 2016;108:332–63. doi: 10.17235/reed.2016.4389/2016

[11] Drossman DA., Hasler WL. Rome IV—Functional GI disorders: disorders of Gut-Brain interaction. Gastroenterology. 2016;150:1257–61. doi: 10.1053/j.gastro.2016.03.035

[12] El-Salhy M. Recent developments in the pathophysiology of irritable bowel syndrome. World J Gastroenterol. 2015;21:7621–36. doi: 10.3748/wjg.v21.i25.7621

[13] El-Salhy M., Gundersen D. Diet in irritable bowel syndrome. Nutr J. 2015;14:36. doi: 10.1186/s12937-015-0022-3

[14] Kellow JE., Miller LJ., Phillips SF., Zinsmeister AR., Charboneau JW. Altered sensitivity of the gallbladder to cholecystokinin octapeptide in irritable bowel syndrome. Am J Physiol. 1987;253:G650–5.

[15] Barbara G., Feinle-Bisset C., Ghoshal UC., Quigley EM., Santos J., Vanner S., Vergnolle N., Zoetendal EG. The intestinal microenvironment and functional gastrointestinal disorders. Gastroenterology. 2016;150:1305–18. doi: 10.1053/j.gastro.2016.02.028

[16] Molina-Infante J., Serra J., Fernandez-Bañares F., Mearin F. The low-FODMAP diet for irritable bowel syndrome: lights and shadows. Gastroenterol Hepatol. 2016;39:55–65. doi: 10.1016/j.gastrohep.2015.07.009

[17] Deng Y., Misselwitz B., Dai N., Fox M. Lactose intolerance in adults: biological mechanism and dietary management. Nutrients. 2015;7:8020–35. doi: 10.3390/nu7095380

[18] Does a low FODMAP diet help IBS? Drug Ther Bull. 2015;53:93–6. doi: 10.1136/dtb.2015.8.0346. http://dtb.bmj.com/content/53/8/93.full.pdf+html.

[19] Gibson PR., Shepherd SJ. Personal view: food for thought - western lifestyle and susceptibility to Crohn's disease. The FODMAP hypothesis. Aliment Pharmacol Ther. 2005;21:1399–409. doi: 10.1111/j.1365-2036.2005.02506.x

[20] Marsh A., Eslick EM., Eslick GD. Does a diet low in FODMAPs reduce symptoms associated with functional gastrointestinal disorders? A comprehensive systematic review and meta-analysis. Eur J Nutr. 2016;55:897–906 doi: 10.1007/s00394-015-0922-1

[21] Fernández-Bañares F., Esteve M., Viver JM. Fructose-sorbitol malabsorption. Curr Gastroenterol Rep. 2009;11:368–74.

[22] Mansueto P., Seidita A., D'Alcamo A., Carroccio A. Role of FODMAPs in patients with irritable bowel syndrome. Nutr Clin Pract. 2015;30:665–82. doi: 10.1177/0884533615569886

[23] Latulippe ME., Skoog SM. Fructose malabsorption and intolerance: effects of fructose with and without simultaneous glucose ingestion. Crit Rev Food Sci Nutr. 2011;51:583–92. doi: 10.1080/10408398.2011.566646

[24] Douard V., Ferraris RP. The role of fructose transporters in diseases linked to excessive fructose intake. J Physiol. 2013;591:401–14. doi: 10.1113/jphysiol.2011.215731

[25] Roberfroid MB. Introducing inulin-type fructans. Br J Nutr. 2005;93(Suppl. 1):S13–25. doi: 10.1079/BJN20041350

[26] Fedewa A., Rao SS. Dietary fructose intolerance, fructan intolerance and FODMAPs. Curr Gastroenterol. 2014;16:370. doi: 10.1007/s11894-013-0370-0

[27] Roberfroid MB., Delzenne NM. Dietary fructans. Annu Rev Nutr. 1998;18:117–43. doi: 10.1146/annurev.nutr.18.1.117

[28] Sangwan V., Tomar SK., Singh RRB., Singh AK., Ali B. Galactooligosaccharides: novel components of designer foods. J Food Sci. 2011;76:R103–11. doi: 10.1111/j. 1750-3841.2011.02131.x

[29] Roberfroid MB. Inulin-type fructans: functional food ingredients. J Nutr. 2007;137:2493S–2502S.

[30] Macfarlane GT., Steed H., Macfarlane S. Bacterial metabolism and health-related effects of galacto-oligosaccharides and other prebiotics. J Appl Microbiol. 2008;104:305–44. doi: 10.1111/j.1365-2672.2007.03520.x

[31] Yao CK., Tan H-L., van Langenberg DR., Barrett JS., Rose R., Liels K., et al. Dietary sorbitol and mannitol: food content and distinct absorption patterns between healthy individuals and patients with irritable bowel syndrome. J Hum Nutr Diet. 2014;27:263–75. doi: 10.1111/jhn.12144

[32] Lomer MCE., Parkes GC., Sanderson JD. Review article: lactose intolerance in clinical practice: myths and realities. Aliment Pharmacol Ther. 2008;27:93–103. doi: 10.1111/j. 1365-2036.2007.03557.x

[33] Swallow DM. Genetics of lactase persistence and lactose intolerance. Annu Rev Genet. 2003;37:197–219. doi: 10.1146/annurev.genet.37.110801.143820

[34] Shaukat A., Levitt MD., Taylor BC., MacDonald R., Shamliyan TA., Kane RL., Wilt TJ. Systematic review: effective management strategies for lactose intolerance. Ann Intern Med. 2010;152:797–803. doi: 10.7326/0003-4819-152-12-201006150-00241

[35] Savaiano DA., Boushey CJ., McCabe GP. Lactose intolerance symptoms assessed by meta-analysis: a grain of truth that leads to exaggeration. J Nutr. 2006;136:1107–13.

[36] Parker TJ., Woolner JT., Prevost AT., Tuffnell Q., Shorthouse M., Hunter JO. Irritable bowel syndrome: is the search for lactose intolerance justified? Eur J Gastroenterol Hepatol. 2001;13:219–25.

[37] Benedé S., Blázquez AB., Chiang D., Tordesillas L., Berin MC. The rise of food allergy: environmental factors and emerging treatments. EBioMedicine. 2016;7:27–34. doi: 10.1016/j.ebiom.2016.04.012

[38] Pasqui F., Poli C., Colecchia A., Marasco G., Festi D. Adverse Food reaction and functional gastrointestinal disorders: role of the dietetic approach. J Gastrointestin Liver Dis. 2015;24:319–27. doi: 10.15403/jgld.2014.1121.243.paq

[39] Ho MH-K., Wong WH-S., Chang C. Clinical spectrum of food allergies: a comprehensive review. Clin Rev Allergy Immunol. 2014;46:225–40. doi: 10.1007/s12016-012-8339-6

[40] Burks AW., Tang M., Sicherer S., Muraro A., Eigenmann PA., Ebisawa M., Fiocchi A., Chiang W., Beyer K., Wood R., Hourihane J., Jones SM., Lack G., Sampson HA. ICON: food allergy. J Allergy Clin Immunol. 2012;129:906–20. doi: 10.1016/j.jaci.2012.02.001

[41] Sampson HA. Food allergy: accurately identifying clinical reactivity. Allergy. 2005;60:19–24. doi: 10.1111/j.1398-9995.2005.00853.x

[42] Caubet J-C., Sampson HA. Beyond skin testing: state of the art and new horizons in food allergy diagnostic testing. Immunol Allergy Clin North Am. 2012;32:97–109. doi: 10.1016/j.iac.2011.11.002

[43] Turnbull JL., Adams HN., Gorard DA. Review article: the diagnosis and management of food allergy and food intolerances. Aliment Pharmacol Ther. 2015;41:3–25. doi: 10.1111/apt.12984

[44] Lieberman JA., Sicherer SH. Diagnosis of food allergy: epicutaneous skin tests, in vitro tests, and oral food challenge. Curr Allergy Asthma Rep. 2011;11:58–64. doi: 10.1007/s11882-010-0149-4

[45] Stiefel G., Roberts G. How to use serum-specific IgE measurements in diagnosing and monitoring food allergy. Arch Dis Child Educ Pract Ed. 2012;97:29–36. doi: 10.1136/archdischild-2011-300569

[46] Siles RI., Hsieh FH. Allergy blood testing: a practical guide for clinicians. Cleve Clin J Med. 2011;78:585–92. doi: 10.3949/ccjm.78a.11023

[47] Bergmann MM., Caubet J-C., Boguniewicz M., Eigenmann PA. Evaluation of food allergy in patients with atopic dermatitis. J Allergy Clin Immunol Pract. 2013;1:22–8. doi: 10.1016/j.jaip.2012.11.005

[48] Makharia A., Catassi C., Makharia GK. The overlap between irritable bowel syndrome and non-celiac gluten sensitivity: a clinical dilemma. Nutrients. 2015;7:10417–26. doi: 10.3390/nu7125541

[49] Di Sabatino A., Corazza GR. Coeliac disease. The Lancet. 2009;373:1480–93. doi: 10.1016/S0140-6736(09)60254-3

[50] Tatham AS., Shewry PR. Allergy to wheat and related cereals. Clin Exp Allergy. 2008;38:1712–26. doi: 10.1111/j.1365-2222.2008.03101.x

[51] Cianferoni A. Wheat allergy: diagnosis and management. J Asthma Allergy. 2016;9:13–25. doi: 10.2147/JAA.S81550

[52] De Giorgio R, Volta U, Gibson PR. Sensitivity to wheat, gluten and FODMAPs in IBS: facts or fiction? Gut. 2016;65:169–78. doi: 10.1136/gutjnl-2015-309757

[53] Biesiekierski JR., Newnham ED., Shepherd SJ., Muir JG., Gibson PR. Characterization of adults with a self-diagnosis of nonceliac gluten sensitivity. Nutr Clin Pract. 2014;29:504–9. doi: 10.1177/0884533614529163

[54] El-Salhy M., Hatlebakk JG., Gilja OH., Hausken T. The relation between celiac disease, nonceliac gluten sensitivity and irritable bowel syndrome. Nutr J. 2015;14:92. doi: 10.1186/s12937-015-0080-6

[55] Biesiekierski JR., Peters SL., Newnham ED., Rosella O., Muir JG., Gibson PR. No effects of gluten in patients with self-reported non-celiac gluten sensitivity after dietary reduction of fermentable, poorly absorbed, short-chain carbohydrates. Gastroenterology. 2013;145:320–8. doi: 10.1053/j.gastro.2013.04.051

[56] Piacentino D., Rossi S., Alvino V., Cantarini R., Badiali D., Pallotta N., et al. Effects of low-FODMAP and gluten-free diets in irritable bowel syndrome patients: a double-blind randomized controlled clinical study. Gastrointest Endosc. 2014;79:S-82. doi: 10.1016/S0016-5085(14)60294-8

[57] Piacentino D., Rossi S., Alvino V., Di Nunno R., Piretta L., Badiali D., et al. 611 Low-FODMAP diet in irritable bowel syndrome patients offers more benefit than a low-FODMAP gluten-free diet in the medium- and long-term: results from a double-blind randomized controlled clinical study and follow-up. Gastroenterology. 2015;148:S-1–S-1196. doi: 10.1016/S0016-5085(15)30414-5

[58] Zanini B., Basché R., Ferraresi A., Ricci C., Lanzarotto F., Marullo M., et al. Randomised clinical study: gluten challenge induces symptom recurrence in only a minority of patients who meet clinical criteria for non-coeliac gluten sensitivity. Aliment Pharmacol Ther. 2015;42:968–76. doi: 10.1111/apt.13372

[59] Molina-Infante J., Santolaria S., Sanders DS., Fernández-Bañares F. Systematic review: noncoeliac gluten sensitivity. Aliment Pharmacol Ther. 2015;41:807–20. doi: 10.1111/apt.13155

[60] Dore J., Simren M., Buttle L., Guarner F. Hot topics in gut microbiota. United Eur Gastroenterol J. 2013;1:311–8. doi: 10.1177/2050640613502477

[61] Power SE., O'Toole PW., Stanton C., Ross RP., Fitzgerald GF. Intestinal microbiota, diet and health. Br J Nutr. 2014;111:387–402. doi: 10.1017/S0007114513002560

[62] Farrugia G., Simren M., Mawe G., Bradesi S., Bredenoord AJ. Gut microbiota and neurogastroenterology and motility: the good the bad and the ugly. Neurogastroenterol Motil. 2014;26:295. doi: 10.1111/nmo.12322

[63] Distrutti E., Monaldi L., Ricci P., Fiorucci S. Gut microbiota role in irritable bowel syndrome: new therapeutic strategies. World J Gastroenterol. 2016;22:2219–41. doi: 10.3748/wjg.v22.i7.2219

[64] Goulet O. Potential role of the intestinal microbiota in programming health and disease. Nutr Rev. 2015;73:32–40. doi: 10.1093/nutrit/nuv039

[65] Bull MJ., Plummer NT. Part 1: the human Gut Microbiome in health and disease. Integr Med Clin J. 2014;13:17–22.

[66] Kellow JE., Azpiroz F., Delvaux M., Gebhart GF., Mertz HR., Quigley EMM., et al. Applied principles of neurogastroenterology: physiology/motility sensation. Gastroenterology. 2006;130:1412–20. doi: 10.1053/j.gastro.2005.08.061

[67] Rinttilä T., Lyra A., Krogius-Kurikka L., Palva A. Real-time PCR analysis of enteric pathogens from fecal samples of irritable bowel syndrome subjects. Gut Pathog. 2011;3:6. doi: 10.1186/1757-4749-3-6

[68] Ponnusamy K., Choi JN., Kim J., Lee S-Y., Lee CH. Microbial community and metabolomic comparison of irritable bowel syndrome faeces. J Med Microbiol. 2011;60:817–27. doi: 10.1099/jmm.0.028126-0

[69] Williams EA., Nai X., Corfe BM. Dietary intakes in people with irritable bowel syndrome. BMC Gastroenterol. 2011;11:9. doi: 10.1186/1471-230X-11-9

[70] Gibson PR., Shepherd SJ. Evidence-based dietary management of functional gastrointestinal symptoms: the FODMAP approach. J Gastroenterol Hepatol. 2010;25:252–8. doi: 10.1111/j.1440-1746.2009.06149.x

[71] Bull MJ., Plummer NT. Part 2: treatments for chronic gastrointestinal disease and gut dysbiosis. Integr Med (Encinitas). 2015;14:25–33.

[72] Rigsbee L., Agans R., Shankar V., Kenche H., Khamis HJ., Michail S., et al. Quantitative profiling of gut microbiota of children with diarrhea-predominant irritable bowel syndrome. Am J Gastroenterol. 2012;107:1740–51. doi: 10.1038/ajg.2012.287

[73] Carroll IM., Ringel-Kulka T., Ferrier L., Wu MC., Siddle JP., Bueno L., et al. Fecal protease activity is associated with compositional alterations in the intestinal microbiota. PLoS One. 2013;8:e78017. doi: 10.1371/journal.pone.0078017

[74] Carroll IM., Ringel-Kulka T., Keku TO., Chang Y-H., Packey CD., Sartor RB., et al. Molecular analysis of the luminal- and mucosal-associated intestinal microbiota in diarrhea-predominant irritable bowel syndrome. AJP Gastrointest Liver Physiol. 2011;301:G799–807. doi: 10.1152/ajpgi.00154.2011

[75] Si J-M., Yu Y-C., Fan Y-J., Chen S-J. Intestinal microecology and quality of life in irritable bowel syndrome patients. World J Gastroenterol. 2004;10:1802–5. doi: 10.3748/WJG.v10.i12.1802

[76] Lee KJ., Tack J. Altered intestinal microbiota in irritable bowel syndrome. Neurogastroenterol Motil. 2010;22:493–8.

[77] Maukonen J. Prevalence and temporal stability of selected clostridial groups in irritable bowel syndrome in relation to predominant faecal bacteria. J Med Microbiol. 2006;55:625–33. doi: 10.1099/jmm.0.46134-0

[78] Balsari A., Ceccarelli A., Dubini F., Fesce E., Poli G. The fecal microbial population in the irritable bowel syndrome. Microbiologica. 1982;5:185–94.

[79] Rajilić-Stojanović M., Jonkers DM., Salonen A., Hanevik K., Raes J., Jalanka J., et al. Intestinal microbiota and diet in IBS: causes, consequences, or epiphenomena? Am J Gastroenterol. 2015;110:278–87. doi: 10.1038/ajg.2014.427

[80] Camilleri M. Serotonin in the gastrointestinal tract. Curr Opin Endocrinol Diabetes Obes. 2009;16:53–9. doi: 10.1097/MED.0b013e32831e9c8e

[81] Halmos EP., Christophersen CT., Bird AR., Shepherd SJ., Gibson PR., Muir JG. Diets that differ in their FODMAP content alter the colonic luminal microenvironment. Gut. 2015;64:93–100. doi: 10.1136/gutjnl-2014-307264

[82] Camilleri M., Lasch K., Zhou W. Irritable bowel syndrome: methods, mechanisms, and pathophysiology: the confluence of increased permeability, inflammation, and pain in irritable bowel syndrome. AJP Gastrointest Liver Physiol. 2012;303:G775–85. doi: 10.1152/ajpgi.00155.2012

[83] Branum AM., Lukacs SL. Food allergy among children in the United States. Pediatrics. 2009;124:1549–55. doi: 10.1542/peds.2009-1210

[84] Berni Canani R., Gilbert JA., Nagler CR. The role of the commensal microbiota in the regulation of tolerance to dietary allergens. Curr Opin Allergy Clin Immunol. 2015;15:243–9. doi: 10.1097/ACI.0000000000000157

[85] Muir AB., Benitez AJ., Dods K., Spergel JM., Fillon SA. Microbiome and its impact on gastrointestinal atopy. Allergy. 2016; 71:1256-63 doi: 10.1111/all.12943.

[86] Halmos EP., Power VA., Shepherd SJ., Gibson PR., Muir JG. A diet low in FODMAPs reduces symptoms of irritable bowel syndrome. Gastroenterology. 2014;146:67–75. doi: 10.1053/j.gastro.2013.09.046

[87] Shepherd SJ., Lomer MCE., Gibson PR. Short-chain carbohydrates and functional gastrointestinal disorders. Am J Gastroenterol. 2013;108:707–17. doi: 10.1038/ajg. 2013.96

[88] Ong DK., Mitchell SB., Barrett JS., Shepherd SJ., Irving PM., Biesiekierski JR., et al. Manipulation of dietary short chain carbohydrates alters the pattern of gas production and genesis of symptoms in irritable bowel syndrome: dietary FODMAPs and IBS symptoms. J Gastroenterol Hepatol. 2010;25:1366–73. doi: 10.1111/j.1440-1746.2010.06370.x

[89] Staudacher HM., Whelan K., Irving PM., Lomer MC. Comparison of symptom response following advice for a diet low in fermentable carbohydrates (FODMAPs) versus standard dietary advice in patients with irritable bowel syndrome. J Hum Nutr Diet. 2011;24:487–95. doi: 10.1111/j.1365-277X.2011.01162

[90] Staudacher HM., Lomer MCE., Anderson JL., Barrett JS., Muir JG., Irving PM., et al. Fermentable carbohydrate restriction reduces luminal bifidobacteria and gastrointestinal symptoms in patients with irritable bowel syndrome. J Nutr. 2012;142:1510–8. doi: 10.3945/jn.112.159285

[91] Böhn L., Störsrud S., Liljebo T., Collin L., Lindfors P., Törnblom H., Simrén M. Diet low in FODMAPs reduces symptoms of irritable bowel syndrome as well as traditional dietary advice: a randomized controlled trialGastroenterology. 2015;149:1399–407.e2. doi: 10.1053/j.gastro.2015.07.054

[92] Koven N., Abry A. The clinical basis of orthorexia nervosa: emerging perspectives. Neuropsychiatr Dis Treat. 2015;11:385–94. doi: 10.2147/NDT.S61665

Chapter 5

Non-Pharmacological Approach to Irritable Bowel Syndrome

Elsa M. Eriksson, Kristina I. Andrén and
Henry T. Eriksson

Additional information is available at the end of the chapter

http://dx.doi.org/10.5772/66373

Abstract

Irritable bowel syndrome (IBS) is a commonly diagnosed gastrointestinal condition. It represents a significant healthcare burden and still remains a real challenge. Over the years, IBS has been described as a strict illness of the gastrointestinal tract (medical model) or as a more complex multi-symptomatic disorder of the brain-gut axis (biopsychosocial or psychosomatic model). The reason why IBS has been such a challenge and is so difficult to handle might be related to different approaches. These differences in the view of the syndrome have affected the assessment, treatment and handling of the IBS patient. Patients with IBS, where the symptoms from the gastrointestinal tract are one part of a multi-symptom palette sometimes hidden in the body or mind, need a more holistic outlook. The key to an effective treatment approach is a gastroenterological examination to exclude other diseases along with an assessment of the whole body and its awareness by a body-mind therapist. This chapter discusses the view of the patient together with patient evaluations and body-mind treatment from a practical point of view.

Keywords: irritable bowel syndrome, body awareness therapy, body-mind evaluation, treatment

1. Introduction

Irritable bowel syndrome (IBS) is one of the most commonly diagnosed gastrointestinal conditions and generates a significant healthcare burden with huge economic costs [1]. In Sweden, 10–20% of the inhabitants suffer from some kind of disturbed bowel function [2]. Many are on long-term sick leave and there are studies showing that about 46% of all sick leaves are due to these patient categories and thus generating high costs for the society [3]. About 30–40% of the patients, consulting healthcare for acute abdominal troubles, are not diagnosed, and hence there might be IBS patients hidden among this group of patients. Increased economic consequences are also incurred as a result of unnecessary surgery. IBS is a common disease with symptoms, including abdominal pain, cramping or bloating. It may also include alteration in bowel habits like faecal urgency or obstipation. Patients may find relief of pain and other discomfort upon defecation. The prevalence of IBS may vary with different definitions and more severe cases can be underestimated. IBS is more prevalent among women. IBS patients can be subdivided in relation to symptoms. The three subtypes are a constipation predominant group (C-IBS), a diarrhoea predominant group (D-IBS) and a group with alternating type (A-IBS) where stool fluctuates between diarrhoea and constipation. In some cases, the symptoms may be so severe that a risk for suicide might occur. A final diagnosis of IBS should be based on clinical symptoms together with exclusion of various somatic diseases [1].

IBS patients often have various other symptoms, beside their gastrointestinal problems. They may have pain in other parts of the body, they may score high psychological symptoms as well as low quality of life. We have also found that they show deviations in body parameters such as body tensions, bodily stress patterns, low body awareness and biochemical stress parameters. Many IBS patients have been subjected to traumatic events and may suffer from a low self-esteem, difficulties setting limits and hypersensitivity. They are often co-diagnosed with fibromyalgia, "burn-out" depression and/or panic disorder. Patients may consult a number of different specialists within gastroenterology (abdominal problems), psychiatry (panic attacks and depression), rheumatology (arthritis), dermatology (eczema and itch) or primary healthcare (chronic fatigue syndrome, fibromyalgia and myalgia). The diagnosis given to a patient with one of these conditions often depends on the characteristic symptoms and the expertise of the treating clinician [1, 2, 4–6].

IBS patients have been reported to have higher levels of stress and more traumatic experiences than patients without gastrointestinal disturbances. Rats, experimentally induced with chronic stress, showed gastrointestinal symptoms (GIS) comparable to IBS. Different parts of the autonomic nervous system (ANS) have been shown to vary in activity when patients display diarrhoea or constipation as pre-dominant symptom of their IBS. When the state of stress continues it may lead to dysfunction of the ANS, that is, an autonomic dysfunction, sometimes called a comprehensive health disturbance. The syndromes in patients with overlapping diagnoses and multi-symptoms have also been called functional somatic syndromes, medically unexplained symptoms, somatoform disorders, unexplained clinical conditions or bodily distress syndrome. It has been suggested that these conditions actually should be gathered under one common name [1–4, 7, 8].

1.1. IBS over the years

The year 1948, Collins defined the syndrome of irritable colon as a "hyperirritable, neuromuscular imbalance of the colon sufficiently severe to cause abdominal pain or distress." He continued that it was "due to functional as well as somatic causes and it is important to emphasise physiologic, local irritative and psychosomatic factors" [9]. In 1956, Bargen wrote "The so called irritable colon is primarily the result of an emotional disturbance, a tension

http://dx.doi.org/10.5772/66373

state, abuse of laxative agents or a dietary indiscretion." Bargen continued "Measures should include particular attention to their emotional disturbances, their situation in respect to stress, and particularly their dietary problems" [10]. IBS was later on (during the 1960s), defined as a disease of the gastrointestinal region with mainly pharmacological treatment. Wessely et al. [11] wrote in 1999 an article entitled "Functional somatic syndromes: one or many?" leading to that several physicians expressed their frustration about the treatment of IBS. Enck and Martens [12] wrote in 2008, "The next consensus for the syndrome of the irritable bowel has to be interdisciplinary." In the late 1970s, the authors started to use the word "biopsychosocial" and up to now about 100 articles have been published according to PubMed using this term in relation to IBS. Throughout the literature, two views emerge, including the medical view of IBS as a strict disease of the gastrointestinal tract, as well as a psychosomatic/biopsychosocial view in which IBS is seen as a complex multi-symptomatic disorder [1].

2. Non-pharmacological treatments

Most research concludes that the management of the complex syndrome IBS should rely on a combination of non-pharmacological and pharmacological therapies with dietary and lifestyle modifications. Some authors claim that treatments involving body and mind are the most effective and powerful treatment strategies in IBS/body distress patients [13–15]. Different non-pharmacological regimens have been used for the treatment of IBS. Body-mind therapies such as gut-directed hypnotherapy, mindfulness therapy, functional relaxation and body awareness therapy have been used with promising results both during treatment and at follow-up. Over the years, treatments have progressed from mostly individual to more group sessions; and there is also a trend towards prolonged sessions. The treatment modalities have also gone from focusing either on the body or the mind to now focusing on both [1].

Hypnotherapy has been used to treat IBS patients with good results since Whorwell et al. introduced it in 1984 [16]. Hypnotherapy means to induce a state of relaxation or trance in response to verbal or other stimuli, with suggestions for improvement made. The patient is taught relaxation, ego strengthening and coping skills. Tailoring the therapy to the patient's symptomatology is essential and the importance of practice is vital and should ideally take place on a daily basis. Hypnotherapy is mostly used with individually tailored technique and 12 sessions of treatment are provided to gain maximum benefit. It has been mostly used with gut-directed therapy; however Carolusson [17] includes both gut-oriented hypnotherapy and hypnoanalysis either separately or in combination. She concludes that hypnosis treatment has to be designed depending on patients' personality and possible mental defence-functions in relation to the symptoms as well as the mental and social resources. This technique is exceptionally operator-dependent; and not suitable for everyone [18]. Whorwell suggests that "hypnotherapy incorporated into a programme with a contingency plan for dealing with individuals who do not respond to this particular form of treatment is the best form of treatment" [19].

To apply *mindfulness* is to practise awareness of internal sensations and to have a non-judgemental approach to all experiences, impressions, thoughts and feelings that comes into awareness and to be fully present in the activities. Gaylord et al. adapted this practice to an IBS population by encouraging the patients to apply this approach on IBS-related symptoms and perceptions. Participants were instructed to notice any sensations in the abdominal area and try to distinguish those sensations from thoughts about the sensations [1, 20].

Functional relaxation is assumed to be a treatment of autonomic dysfunction with proprioception and a part of body awareness. During relaxed expiration, very subtle movements of the small joints are performed, when at the same time, the patient, focus and explore the perceived body sensations which are triggered by the movements. This takes unconscious body-mind experiences into account and, due to rediscovery and development of basic motivational systems, previously forgotten forms of bodily self-awareness can be re-experienced [1, 21].

Body awareness therapy (BAT™) is structured movements based on human anatomical and physiological requirements to achieve optimal dynamics. The BAT™ alludes to help the body find its natural posture. Then the body systems (circular, muscular, nerves and breathing) facilitate to recover their natural function. By doing so, unconscious body and mind experiences can come into awareness. Practising body awareness includes presence, reflection and acceptance. BAT™ was developed in Sweden by physiotherapists in the early 1970s. Nowadays it is used for treatment of various stress and pain-related conditions in all Nordic countries, as well as in Estonia, Austria, Scotland, Switzerland, the Netherlands, Spain and Turkey [1, 22].

One common point of these methods is training on how to be in the here and now; to be aware of the present. Body-mind training affects the level of muscular tension, the posture, the breathing, together with the function and mobility of the inner organs. The bodily experiences always exist in the present, and the awareness of emotions is inseparable from the consciousness of their bodily expressions. Altogether, these express how a person feels mentally and physically. In this way, these therapies, embracing body and mind, are assumed to work through a physiological transformation accomplished via the ANS [21, 23]. Although the methods differ slightly in how they are addressed, either through the mind (hypnotherapy or mindfulness) or through the body (body awareness therapy or functional relaxation), the treatment results are similar [1].

3. The Studies of Functional Bowel Syndrome and Treatment (SOFT) project

A project was started in 2000 with the purpose of examining patients with functional bowel disorders and compare them with healthy volunteers (without bowel disorders), and further to evaluate the effects of body awareness therapy on the patients symptoms. Since 2004, the authors (KA, gestalt therapist/BSc in chemistry/biomedicine and EE, physiotherapist/PhD in biochemistry/physiology, both trained and certified in BAT) have worked together and treated approximately 340 patients. Patients are referred from both primary and special care units (medicine and surgery), about 30% from each. Due to IBS being such a complex syndrome and our diversified backgrounds, we were interested in evaluating as many symptoms as possible reported by the patients. In a smaller study of IBS patients, vitamins, fatty acids and minerals were followed. We have also tried to characterise the IBS subtypes according to the data measured. In an epidemiologic study including a random population sample from the general population in Gothenburg, Sweden, we studied the correlation of gastrointestinal symptoms to other symptomatology in the same population. The SOFT studies and their results are described on the following sections. For practical reasons, the IBS patient is referred to as a women (she) in the following text.

3.1. The examination procedure in the SOFT study

After a thorough interview including medical history and their narrated experience, the patients are examined with two physical examinations: a resource-oriented body examination (ROBE) and a moving test body awareness scale-health (BAS-H) (**Table 1**). The ROBE examination evaluates body posture, function, respiration, passive mobility, balance and muscular degree of palpation. BAS-H evaluates grounding, midline, respiration and ability to set limits. The BAS-H test is based upon observations made by a physiotherapist of defined items on basic movements (BASobs) as well as standardised questions concerning their body awareness (BASself). From these two examinations one can get a picture of, to what degree the patient herself is aware of her body and its tensions. Patients in the project complete self-assessment questionnaires concerning psychological and psychosocial symptoms, pain, bodily symptoms and also a questionnaire regarding gastrointestinal symp-

Anamnesis	
Psychosomatic physiotherapeutic examinations	
	Resource-oriented body examination (ROBE)
	Body awareness scale examination (BAS-H)
Blood and saliva samples	
	Cortisol, prolactin, C-peptide, TG (triglycerides), minerals
	Vitamins
Questionnaires	
	GIS (Gastro Intestinal Scale, gastrointestinal symptoms)
	SCL90 (Symptom Check List 90, general symptoms, rating how much)
	CS (Complaint scale, general symptoms, rating how often)
	SOC (sense of coherence, health concepts related to quality of life)
	PRS (psychosocial rating scale)
Pain body map	Women/man
Food diary	4 days (including Saturday and Sunday)

Table 1. Examinations of the patients in the SOFT project.

toms. The CS scale measures autonomic dysfunction and can be divided into a vegetative, muscular and psychological part. Stress parameters in blood and saliva are also measured [1, 4–6].

In our study, the patients are evaluated at the unit two to three times during a total time of approximately 3 h, before starting treatment. After these examinations and meetings, we can form an opinion of each patient and what she may need to reduce symptoms and improve quality of life. These procedures also give us a hint of to what extent the patient is able to comply with our group treatment, and if we need to strengthen and support her regarding this before the start of treatment. Individual dialogues are held and questionnaires are completed at four times, one before treatment, one after 12 and 24 weeks, respectively, and also 6 months after the end of treatment.

3.2. The subtype study

Eighty IBS patients (30 D-IBS, 16 C-IBS and 34 A-IBS) underwent physiotherapeutic examinations (for dysfunctions in body movements/awareness) and were compared to an apparently healthy control group. Both IBS patients and controls answered questionnaires regarding psychological (SCL90) and gastrointestinal symptoms. Biochemical variables were analysed in blood. The subtypes were compared with each other and the control group [6].

3.3. The mineral, vitamin and fatty acids study

In a sub-study, 30 IBS patients were analysed for whole blood or serum levels of vitamins (B6, B12, E, Q10 and folic acid), minerals (Na, K, Ca, Mg, Cu, Fe, P, PB, Li, Zn and Selenium) and fatty acids (saturated, mono-unsaturated, Ω3 and Ω6). Questionnaires for gastrointestinal symptoms (GIS) and psychological symptoms (SCL90) were completed and correlated. Results from questionnaires versus minerals were calculated. The patients were grouped according to reference ranges established by the laboratory (Lab. für spektralanalytische und biologische Untersuchungen, Stuttgart, Germany) [24].

3.4. The epidemiologic study

The study of "Men born 1913" started in Gothenburg in 1963. In 2003, women born 1953 were included for the first time and a total of 668 women of 50 years old were randomly selected from the general population. We focused on gastrointestinal symptoms such as "have you during the last three months suffered from diarrhoea and/or constipation." The women were extensively screened with examinations such as descriptive data (body weight, height, BMI, waist hip, circumference, smoking and alcohol), somatic data (blood pressure, cholesterol, triglycerides, glucose and diseases) and vegetative data such as (dizziness, perspiration, breathlessness, indisposition and chilliness). Additionally, questions regarding stress were included (experience of stress, burnout and absence from work due to stress), psychological expression (lack of sleep, nervous symptom and easily moved to tears), psychosocial symptoms (situation of work, home, economics, health, memory and energy), grade of occupation (work, sick list and early pension) and medication were registered [25, 26].

4. Results

4.1. Before treatment evaluation of IBS patients in the SOFT study

Before treatment, evaluations show that IBS patients have deviated movement patterns, for example, grounding, midline, centration, setting up limits and awareness of respiration (BAS-H). Further they may have an impact on posture, body function (flexibility, spontaneous movement and passive activity), respiration and the muscular system (ROBE). Stress-parameters in blood and saliva can be affected and some patients also have mineral and vitamin deficiencies. Furthermore, they often present a low quality of life, and in many cases have experienced traumatic events (such as bullying in school, parental premature death, sexual abuse, war experiences or violations by the healthcare). They may also have psychological symptoms and autonomic dysfunction. The IBS patient thus shows many signs of being in a chronic condition of strain. In other words – they have an internal stress. Patients may have difficulties with trusting healthcare providers. Several patients have been adversely affected by previous visits. Often they have been told: "This is stress you will have to live with"; "With positive thinking it will be better." They often feel wrecked and angry, and tell that they have lost their self-confidence and self-esteem [1, 3–6].

When assessed before treatment, the patients in our study showed mostly deviated patterns in the results from the gastrointestinal survey, the body-oriented examinations and the pain drawings, in contrast to the psychological and biochemical data which were within normal limits or deviated (**Table 2**). From our experience to date, none of the patient from more than 300 patients have expressed only gastrointestinal symptoms [1, 3].

4.2. Results subtype study

The IBS patients as a whole group, as well as divided into subtypes, show higher triglyceride values compared to controls. When the material is divided into subtypes, the D-IBS group differ from the other two subtypes with significantly higher C-peptide values and lower prolactin values. This group score an almost normal degree in the questionnaire of sense of coherence (SOC) and thus showed a good quality of life. This was also reflected from the

Parts	Comments
Body oriented (ROBE, BAS-H)	Deviating in most cases
Pain (bodymap)	Deviating in most cases
Psychological (questionnaires)	Deviating or normal
Biochemical (blood, saliva)	Deviating or normal

Table 2. General results from examinations of IBS-patients.

D-IBS patients in a less distorted psychosocial rating scale in comparison with the other two subtypes. However, they express a high pain score similar to the other subtypes. The D-IBS group shows a disturbed body movement pattern on BASobs of the same magnitude as that of the C-IBS and the A-IBS group. However, on self-estimation (BASself) they rate themselves as having less dysfunction (not in conformity with the rating of the physiotherapist) reflecting a lower sense of body awareness. Compared to C-IBS and A-IBS, the D-IBS has the same amount of gastrointestinal symptoms but less psychological symptoms.

The C-IBS patients have higher prolactin values both compared to the controls and the D-IBS subtype. To some extent, similar pattern is seen in the C-IBS and the A-IBS group. On BASself examination both C-IBS and A-IBS rate themselves at the same level as did the physiotherapist. Both these subtypes suffer from more psychological and gastrointestinal symptoms, than was seen among controls. And the C-IBS patients have more psychological symptoms than the A-IBS group. Both groups display a lower quality of life outlined in the psychosocial rating scale and in the sense of coherence scale. Besides, they are afflicted with higher pain scores compared to the controls.

4.3. Results mineral study

IBS patients show considerable deficiencies of predominant minerals in whole blood. The study shows that only a small number of the tested IBS patients have levels within reference ranges (**Figure 1**). Values, both above and below the reference range (outliers), correlate to both gastrointestinal and psychological symptoms. Mineral values within reference ranges correspond to less gastrointestinal symptoms, both totally (Mg**, Cu* and Ca*) and for the sub-items gastrointestinal pain (Mg**), nausea (Ca*) and motility (Mg* and Ca*), see example for Ca (**Figure 2**). Mineral values within reference ranges correspond to less psychological symptoms as seen for Zink (**Figure 3**). These mineral shortages can contribute to the symptom map of the IBS patient. For the other substances measured more individual patterns are seen.

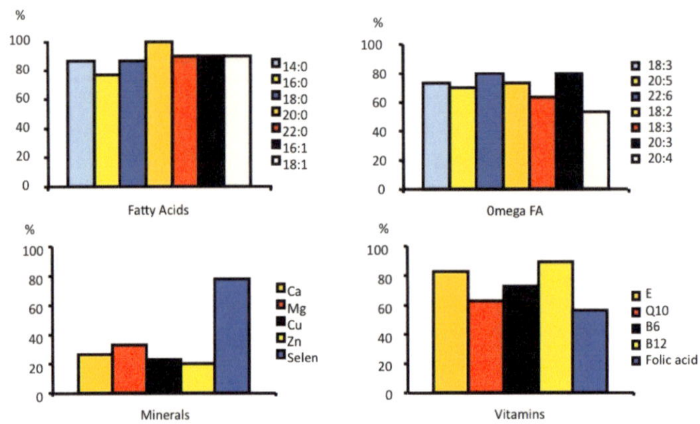

Figure 1. Percentage within reference ranges* for vitamins, minerals and fatty acids. *Lab. für spektralanalytische und biologische untersuchungen, Stuttgart, Germany.

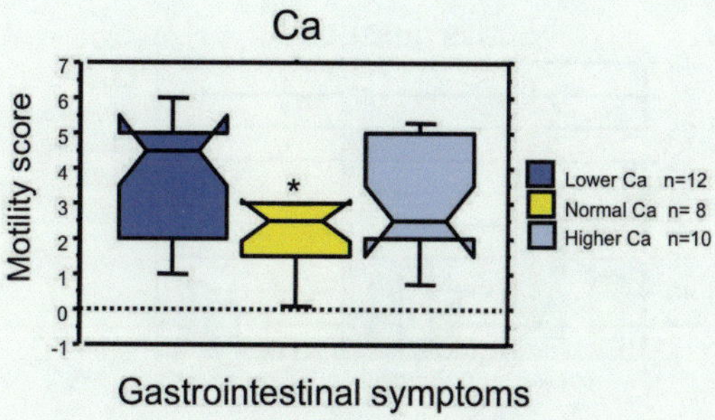

Figure 2. IBS patients with Ca levels within reference ranges express less gastro-intestinal symptoms, here illustrated as motility score. "Motility" = sensation of incomplete evacuation, sensation of urge to defecate. The higher score the more symptoms.

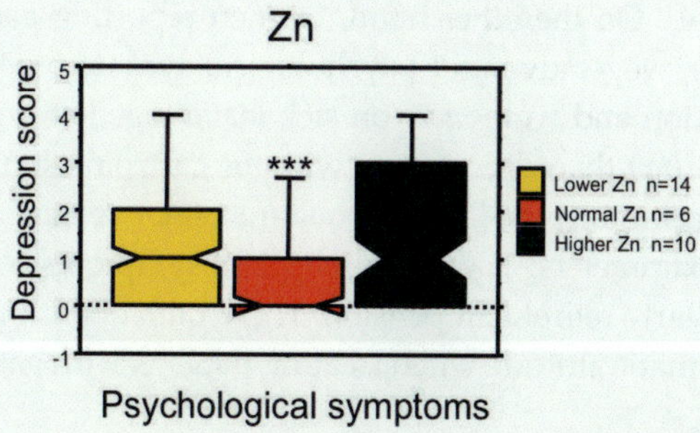

Figure 3. IBS patients with Zn levels within reference ranges express less psychological symptoms, here illustrated as depressive score. "Depression"—feelings of energy loss, suicidal ideation, easily crying and feeling—captured, lonely, depressed, anxious, hopeless or worthless. The higher score the more symptoms.

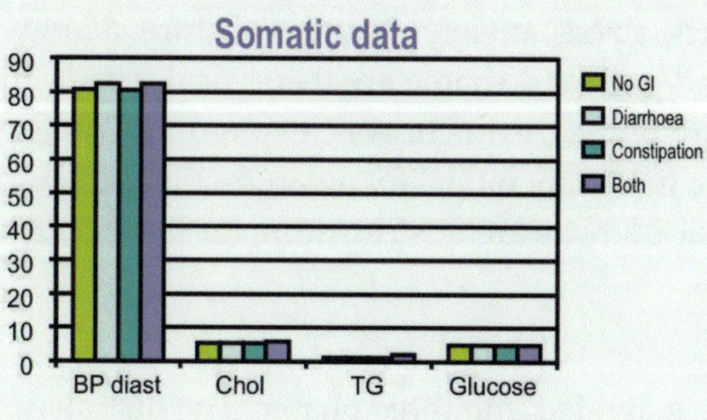

Figure 4. Score for some somatic data for the control group and the GI groups (diarrhoea, constipation and both).

4.4. Results epidemiologic study

Totally 668 of 994 invited 50-year-old women participated in the study. Of these 668 examined women, 492 (73.7%) had no gastrointestinal symptom. A total of 64 women (9.6%) reported diarrhoea, 85 (12.7%) stated constipation and 27 (4%) reported a mixture of diarrhoea and

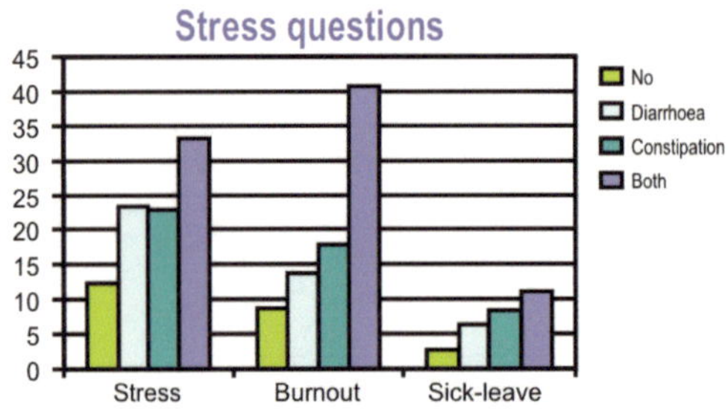

Figure 5. Score for stress, burnout and sick leave for the control group and the GI groups (diarrhoea, constipation and both).

constipation. No significant differences were seen between the controls (*no gastrointestinal problems*) and those women with gastrointestinal symptoms regarding *any of* the descriptive or somatic data (**Figure 4**). On the other hand, women reporting gastrointestinal symptoms showed significantly *more* vegetative and psychological symptoms, felt *more* stressed, had a *worse* psychosocial situation and were *more* on sick leave together with maintaining sickness pension in a *higher proportion* than did women without gastrointestinal symptoms (**Figure 5**). Our study shows that gastrointestinal symptoms are rather related to stress and psychosomatics, than to somatic parameters. The gastrointestinal symptoms contribute to an increased degree of sick leave and early retirement pension. These data underline the importance of considering *a more* psychosomatic attitude when treating patients with gastrointestinal symptoms.

5. The treatment procedure in the SOFT study

Process-oriented treatment is given in the form of body awareness practice in groups (8–12 individuals), 2 h per time on 24 occasions. Each occasion consists of bodily practice, theory and reflection. Psychosomatics, stress, anxiety, trauma, posture, allergy, IBS, food, body awareness, self-image, ANS and guilt and shame are theoretical themes that are addressed during each course. The structure of the treatment was inspired by Torrestad et al. [27], who developed a physiotherapeutic treatment model for awareness and relaxation. The bodily exercises derived mainly from basic body awareness (Institute for Basic Body awareness IBK™) [22].

5.1. The structure

Generally, the treatment is divided into three phases. The first phase is all about the body, its needs and body awareness. In the second phase, focus lies on changing the bodily behaviour. During the third part the training is aimed to integrate new insights and changes in everyday life. The same basic exercises are used each time; they are carried out easily from the beginning and are gradually expanded. Other exercises are included, if necessary. The focus lies on practicing body awareness, that is, to be aware of what is happening in the body. The order between lying, sitting, standing and walking exercises is varied in accordance with the group process. Most of the exercises can be performed in ways that are more stabilising or opening, and depending on the reaction of the patients, the exercises can be individually adjusted by the therapists. Every meeting begins and ends with a reflective discussion, in which each participant says her name and possibly something about how the past week has been, and how the body is feeling and at the end of the meeting, what has been noticed in the body during today's class.

5.2. The role of the leaders

Before each class the leaders outline a programme for the day which is adapted to the group process, focusing on the resources of the patients. Leaders keep diary on how the exercises are working and about themes that are expressed in the discussions. These notes created together with the leaders' own reflections, a basis for planning and the next training session. The purpose is to mediate the knowledge, both practical and theoretical, that each individual need in her process towards a better health. This purpose is reflected in the leaders' approach to the patients' questions and comments, as well as in planning the exercises and the theory.

6. The treatment results in the SOFT study

In conclusion, the studies in the SOFT project show that as the patients' gastrointestinal symptoms decrease, their pain decreases, they feel better and experience less anxiety and depression. They develop better relations to their own body and to the life around them. Patients change from having a feeling of being controlled by their gut and their symptoms to feeling safer and to be able to handle different situations in life, both physically and mentally. This treatment affects the patients' body, their feelings, thoughts and actions (**Table 3**).

6.1. Body examinations

ROBE shows that patients improve the variable function during treatment. They are also more relaxed and develop a higher degree of body awareness and a more normalised tension pattern at muscle palpation. In the BAS-H (the movement part of BAS-H), the IBS patients showed improvements. IBS patients also expressed awareness (the interview part of BAS-H) of their improvements, particularly in relation to the ground and in centring of the movements but also to breathing, and to the ability to set limits [3–5].

6.2. Surveys, SCL90, CS and SOC

Psychological symptoms at baseline scored with SCL90 were significantly more common in the IBS group than in the healthy control group. IBS patients score lower levels of psychological symptoms such as depression, obsession, paranoid ideation, anxiety, phobic anxiety and psychoticism after treatment, as measured by SCL90. The items of depression and somatisation were positively correlated. Patients show improvements in the vegetative part of the CS scale early in the treatment period (at the 12 weeks assessment) which then continued. The IBS patients showed a lower sense of coherence than the controls

I have noticed:	
"Body"	*how I am sitting, standing and walking, and if I am anxious or relaxed*
	that feelings quickly transmit to the stomach
"Mind"	*that I am better in expressing my needs, and how I want to do things without bullying others and when I am assertive, I get positive response and people listen to me*
I have started thinking about:	
"Body"	*to recognise when the stress in the body speeds up (to stop in time),*
	I respect more than previously how the body is feeling
	myself, I feel safe to listen to my body
"Mind"	*my past and how it has affected me*
	to take it easy, to cool down
	to not care so much about what other people think about me
I have started to change	
"Body"	*I have great use of the exercises that I learned at our meetings; I practice them daily and have now only minor phases of pain from the diverticulums*
	I feel more vitality and joy in my body.
"Mind"	*my ideas of achievement/performance, I don't have to do everything so much better than everyone else anymore*
	my way of interacting with others, I stand up for myself and my needs and I am, at the same time, more sensitive for the need of the other

Table 3. Patients' comments after 24 weeks of treatment.

before treatment. There were also differences in the items of comprehensibility, manageability and meaningfulness. Their sense of coherence or coping ability shows improvement during the treatment period in total and for each subtype. Before treatment, some patients scored themselves very low, comparable to levels reported from patients who had tried to commit suicide.

6.3. Pain drawings

At baseline, pain drawing gives higher scores for IBS patients than for healthy controls. In addition to pain in the stomach, IBS patients also have other bodily pain of different qualities, for example, in shoulders, arms, back, breast, head, leg and foot. No difference is seen between the subtypes (D-IBS, C-IBS and A-IBS) in this respect and the pain gradually decreased with treatment [3–5].

http://dx.doi.org/10.5772/66373

6.4. Saliva cortisol

Measurements of saliva cortisol indicate that IBS patients can be classified into two groups according to how cortisol levels are reflected in the saliva during the day (diurnal cortisol). One group showed increased diurnal slope and another group lower diurnal slope, which may be interpreted as "overstressed" and "burnt out," respectively. Diurnal cortisol went towards normalisation after treatment with BAT, irrespective of the starting levels. Somatic symptoms correlated with biochemical symptoms. There was a correlation between the most normal score of muscle palpation and a more optimal slope of saliva cortisol [6].

6.5. Observations during treatment

In our study, we as leaders have recurrently noted indications that patients become more grounded and more relaxed during treatment. We observe, for example, better balance in movements and decreased facial tension. The patients develop a better relationship with their own bodies, which, for example, is noticeable when they find it easier to relate to their own body and express more positive opinions about it. They also score lower levels of psychological symptoms after treatment. As the patients become more aware of their symptoms, they improve their body awareness and their symptoms decrease. In the group situation, the changes are also reflected. For example, patients who are very silent when treatment starts will gradually become more confident and start talking more in the group, and those who early on, do not take part in pair exercises will later on join these exercises. Other patients reported that they no longer are dwelling on injustices in the past, and now could let them go and move on forward in their lives [3–5].

7. Working relationship between patient and therapist

Many authors emphasise the importance of a good working treatment relationship between the patient and the therapist/clinician. In order to get an optimal treatment, the therapists need to explore how to create practicable channels of contact. A person with a cognitive orientation wants to obtain a theoretically plausible explanation of her problems in order to feel safe and secure. A person with alexithymia, who cannot express and do not have words for her emotions, needs to increase her body awareness, in order to become comfortable with her body. A person with a vivid and colourful imagination is probably receptive to exercises that include mental visualisation. An optimal treatment plan should comprise all of these components [1].

7.1. Aspects of performing body-mind therapies

When treating IBS patients, who has tendency to dissociate, the therapist must be careful not to re-victimise the patient and thus risk the patient dropping out. By noticing early warning signs for dissociation and with careful guidance, the patients can learn how to build a trusting relationship with themselves and others, in order to maintain both a psychological and a physical integrity (setting up limits) and also to facilitate for the patients to find words to describe the body-signals and sensations. With increasing body awareness, the patients will learn how to stabilise themselves when emotional systems are aroused. In order to first perceive the body and then to connect the sensations in the body with a certain sense or emotion is crucial for the treatment to be effective. The patient may express after several treatment sessions: "Before I just had a stomach ache, but now it is like that just before I get pain, I feel angry" [1, 3].

7.2. Duration of body-mind treatment

The length of treatment can be crucial [1]. Short treatment duration is not always sufficient for all patients; some can be left behind as they display more symptoms. In our studies we have found different patient treatment processes. IBS patients grade themselves on different symptom questionnaires, and both body and biochemical parameters are evaluated; the process can be determined by such parameters. For example, one patient can estimate high levels of symptoms before treatment that are reduced after treatment. Another patient might start by estimating low levels before treatment and score higher at 12 weeks and then lower again after 24 weeks. Such a patient probably need more time to become aware of her bodily sensations, and thus "underestimated" the levels of her symptoms/sensations before the treatment start. A third patient can score increasing symptoms throughout the entire treatment period. This example shows a patient who started out with having a substantially low body awareness, whose experiences have been out of reach/hidden in the body and then slowly arouse into awareness during the treatment process. Hence, treatment of this patient should not be concluded until the patient's symptoms decrease [1, 3–6].

8. Discussion

Many authors, including Collins et al. [9], Bargen [10] and Enck et al. [12], have stressed that IBS is a complicated condition with both physiological and psychological factors involved in the pathogenesis [1]. Moser points out that in practice, functional gastrointestinal disorders are the most frequent disorder seen and suggest that integrated psychosomatic care should be provided [28]. This is in line with the results from our SOFT project with physical, psychological and biochemical examinations and treatment of the "whole person" using body awareness therapy.

The SOFT study has shown that as the patients' gastrointestinal symptoms decreases, the pain decreases, they feel better and experience less depression and anxiety. The patients express a greater awareness of their own potential to affect their symptoms and are more able to control their lives. They change from feeling controlled by their gut and their symptoms to feel safer and able to handle different situations in life, both physically and mentally. Other studies confirm that patients' gastrointestinal symptoms and the extra-intestinal manifestations improve along with increased body awareness [1, 3].

Levels of anxiety and depression are significantly higher among patients with IBS in comparison with apparently healthy persons without IBS [7, 9, 10]. Something that may contrib-

http://dx.doi.org/10.5772/66373

ute to the reduction in health-related quality of life in patients with IBS is the ability to cope with stressful circumstances in life. Antonovsky [29] says that a person needs a strong sense of coherence (SOC) to be able to cope with significant life stressor. Patients having alternating constipation and diarrhoea may be a great problem of daily life that could be considered highly stressful. Thus, a strong SOC might lessen the impact of various stressors on well-being or the stressors themselves can weaken SOC. Motzer et al. [30] have searched for therapeutic ways to increase SOC and quality of life and thus ease the psychological distress associated with IBS. Sperber et al. [31] questioned whether SOC represent a predictor of treatment success or is an outcome variable (which is changeable). We believe that SOC can act both as a predictor and an outcome variable. A low SOC may be a predictor at baseline reflecting the severity of IBS, and thus could prolong the duration of treatment (predictor). However, in the end of the study patients altered their sense of coherence (outcome variable) towards normality values as a result of the therapy [5].

Saliva cortisol in healthy persons has straight downward slopes during daytime. A more negative stress response is reflected by a lower saliva cortisol slope and is an indicator of accumulated physiological and psychosocial stress [32]. A lower slope associated with too high or too low muscle palpation grade was seen in our study. An increased slope of saliva cortisol belonged for the most part to the group with a somewhat increased muscle palpation grade. An increased slope may represent the first phase of the body trying to compensate for stress while a lower slope represents chronic stress and/or exhaustion [33]. Saliva cortisol in the IBS patients changed during treatment; both the lower and the increased slope approached the slope of the controls.

From the SOFT subtype study, it seems the D-IBS patients differ from the other subtypes. D-IBS patients, with a higher proportion of men, scored less psychological symptoms, less body awareness, but scored a better sense of coherence and showed higher C-peptide values in blood. They were not aware of their lack of body awareness and did not realise entirely their depreciated state of health. Overall, they showed themselves to be ambitious persons, and there were more men compared to the other subtypes. Also, many of them were in the middle of their professional careers. The higher C-peptide and triglyceride levels may be parts of a metabolic syndrome, which is known to correlate with psychosocial stress possibly indicating an adrenergic onset that could represent an unconscious mental stress. When studying predominant symptoms in IBS and correlation with autonomic nervous system deviations it was found that the D-IBS subgroup was associated with adrenergic nervous system malfunctions. Prolactin may be important in the process of coping with stress and traumatic experience and it has been reported that active soldiers have lower prolactin values. A strong correlation has been shown between prolactin and alexithymia especially the item "difficulty to identifying feelings." The D-IBS group in our study had both lower prolactin values and lower body awareness [6].

The C-IBS and A-IBS patients are characterised by their psychological symptoms, with more depression and anxiety and with impaired sense of coherence. They express higher degree of body awareness compared to the D-IBS group. Emotional strain and an increased vagal tone are correlated to increased levels of prolactin which could be one reason for the measured prolactin increase in the C-IBS group [6]. Although the sample size of the present study of subtypes is fairly modest, all subjects were recruited from patients with rather advanced IBS disease with several years' history of symptoms. Since they were referred from various doctors from different clinics they could represent a general population of IBS patients.

According to Gonsalkorale et al. [34], IBS has gained the reputation of being somewhat unrewarding to treat. As a consequence, many physicians although performing thorough examinations ensure their patients that there are nothing seriously wrong but offer no remedy to treat the condition. Many patients, especially those who have had their troublesome symptoms for a long time have lost their confidence and feel like "failures" with no hope when they enter our study [1]. Dysregulation of the autonomic nervous system and the emotional system can involve reactions in which the distress inside the body is not recognised because of location or due to low body awareness. This may be one explanation why patients have difficulty identifying their symptoms and can contribute to the fact that there might be misunderstandings between the IBS patients and healthcare providers [1, 3–6]. Another possible explanation could be the two different views of IBS, as mentioned earlier; when the treating doctor views IBS as a strict gastrointestinal disease he will be more apt to a reassuring approach. On the other hand, the doctor who embraces the view that IBS is a more complex disorder will refer the patient to a competent body-mind therapist or a multi-professional team offering a more psychosomatic therapy.

As IBS patients express a great deal of symptoms, they often find themselves somewhat lost within the normal healthcare system with its specialisation. For example, within the field of gastroenterology, some hospitals have various departments for the upper and lower gastrointestinal tract. This involves a great risk that the patients with multiple symptoms and multiple diagnoses are inadequately treated since their cases fall in between different categories [1, 3]. When practising a team approach to management with a graduated treatment programme, extremely high levels of satisfaction in patients and in staff can be achieved [34]. As we saw in the epidemiologic study of 50-year-old women, gastrointestinal symptoms were common in that population and showed a strong correlation to psychosomatic symptoms. Therefore, a more psychosomatic attitude in diagnosis and treatment of these women might have great impact on their well-being.

Many authors stress the importance of a thorough examination of IBS patients with their many symptoms after having excluded important somatic diseases. In the SOFT project, the comprehensive body examination gave us a hint about the treatment duration needed for the patient to improve. When IBS patients are receiving too short treatment duration, the patient may experience relief from some symptoms, but with the underlying distress still present, they will remain untreated and symptoms can be replaced by other symptoms (known as a symptom shift). In these cases, there is a risk that the patients will continue to seek treatment elsewhere and thus get caught between specialities and might never come to understand their internal body mind communication [17]. Patients who need longer treatment periods could be patients that can be defined as non-responders, males with D-IBS, fibromyalgia patients or those who have severe social stress; all factors are likely to cause detraction from the efficacy of the treatment.

http://dx.doi.org/10.5772/66373

Hypnotherapy, mindfulness treatment and body awareness therapy will almost certainly improve the patients' coping skills in various life situations. These methods involve the body by normalising tension, and they also emphasise the importance of being present in the moment. It is only in the present time that you can access and influence the experience and behaviour patterns, which are established in the nervous system [35]. A plausible consequence of this is that consciousness of the "here and now" is very substantial for changing the processes and should be the focus of therapy from the beginning. The habits of non-optimal movement and tension patterns, whether due to chronic stress or other mechanisms, can become so established in the body that you are incapable of changing them on your own. These habits are integrated as part of the self-perception and can be unconsciously hidden together with other suppressed feelings and tensions. To deal with ingrained muscular pattern, the patients must be re-educated and trained until the new patterns feel at least equally familiar as the old ones [36]. Paradoxically, patients need body awareness training to be aware of their tensed bodies before they can start to change and in a deeper sense learn to apply the body awareness therapy [1, 3]. The body awareness technique can thus be used to take control of unwanted symptoms and to reduce psychological distress and improve coping skills [1, 3].

9. Conclusion

From the SOFT project it can be concluded that IBS patients, in comparison with healthy controls have higher degree of body tension and gastrointestinal and psychological symptoms and also biochemical stress markers compared to healthy controls. Our treatment with body awareness therapy reduced these parameters and helped these multi-symptomatic patients feel better. This treatment can be practised for all types of IBS, and since it is performed in groups it is therefore suitable for treating quite a large number of patients at the same time. Our structure of treatment in the SOFT study, combining bodily exercises with theoretical reflections and including time for reflexions in the group, has proven to be beneficial for our patients.

The future health problems are generally considered to be of psychosomatic or psychosocial nature. This should cause us great concern, and we need a new approach for these multi-symptomatic patients and not least the IBS patients. Good teamwork is important during this new approach to treat multi-symptom patients. Therapists/physicians should talk to each other about IBS cases and/or work in a team to ensure that any real or potential problem that may arise can be promptly resolved. When planning effective treatment strategies it is of utmost importance to understand the diversity of this syndrome. Thus, treatment should be aimed at body-mind intervention after having performed a good evaluation survey of each patient both by a gastroenterologist and a body-mind therapist. The duration of treatment should be individually adjusted. Following the same patients systematically, before, during and after treatment seems to be the best method of choice at present. These patients need a psychosomatic approach which is emphasised from our epidemiologic study. Applying a more psychosomatic attitude when diagnosing and treating these patients will give a more optimal caring and in the long run lowered medical healthcare costs.

Author details

Elsa M. Eriksson*, Kristina I. Andrén and Henry T. Eriksson

*Address all correspondence to: elsa.eriksson@surgery.gu.se

Department of Functional Gastroenterology, Sahlgrenska University Hospital, Göteborg, Sweden

References

[1] Eriksson EM, Andrén KI, Kurlberg GK, Eriksson HT. Aspects of the non-pharmacological treatment of irritable bowel syndrome. *World J Gastroenterol* 2015; **21**: 11439–11449. DOI:10.3748/wjg.v21.i40.11439. Review.

[2] Ålander T, Svärdsudd K, Agréus L. Functional gastrointestinal disorder is associated with increased non-gastrointestinal healthcare consumption in the general population. *Int J Clin Pract* 2008; **62**: 234–240. DOI:10.1111/j.1742-1241.2007.01549.x

[3] Biguet G, Keskinen-Rosenqvist R, Levy-Berg A. Understanding the body's message – approaches from the physiotherapists' point of view. 1st ed. Lund: Studentlitteratur, 2012. ISBN:9789144073217

[4] Eriksson E, Nordwall V, Kurlberg G, Rydholm H. Effects of body awareness therapy in patients with irritable bowel syndrome. *Adv Physiol Educ* 2002; **4**: 125–135. DOI:10.1080/140381902320387540

[5] Eriksson EM, Möller IE, Söderberg RH, Eriksson HT, Kurlberg GK. Body awareness therapy: a new strategy for relief of symptoms in irritable bowel syndrome patients. *World J Gastroenterol* 2007; **13**: 3206–3214. PMID: 17589899 DOI:10.3748/WJG.v13.i23.3206

[6] Eriksson EM, Andrén KI, Eriksson HT, Kurlberg GK. Irritable bowel syndrome subtypes differ in body awareness, psychological symptoms and biochemical stress markers. *World J Gastroenterol* 2008; **14**: 4889–4896. PMID: 18756596 DOI:10.3748/wjg.14.4889

[7] White DL, Savas LS, Daci K, Elserag R, Graham DP, Fitzgerald SJ, Smith SL, Tan G, El-Serag HB. Trauma history and risk of irritable bowel syndrome in women veterans. *Aliment Pharmacol Ther* 2010; **32**: 551–561. DOI:10.1111/j.1365-2036.2010.04387.x

[8] Vicario M, Guilarte M, Alonso C, Yang P, Martínez C, Ramos L, Lobo B, González A, Guilà M, Pigrau M, Saperas E, Azpiroz F, Santos J. Chronological assessment of mast cell-mediated gut dysfunction and mucosal inflammation in a rat model of chronic psychological stress. *Brain Behav Immun* 2010; **24**: 1166–1175. DOI:10.1016/j.bbi.2010.06.002

[9] Collins EN. The diagnosis and treatment of irritable colon; physiologic, local irritative and psychosomatic factors. *Med Clin North Am* 1948; **32**: 398–407. PMID:18902879

[10] Bargen JA. The problem of the syndrome of irritable bowel. *Gastroenterology* 1956; **30**: 703–706. PMID:13318254

[11] Wessely S, Nimnuan C, Sharpe M. Functional somatic syndromes: one or many? *Lancet* 1999; **354**: 936–939. DOI:10.1016/S0140-6736(98)08320-2

[12] Enck P, Martens U. The next consensus for the irritable bowel syndrome has to be interdisciplinary. *Z Gastroenterol* 2008; **46**: 211–215. DOI:10.1055/s-2007-963341

[13] Fink P, Schröder A. One single diagnosis, bodily distress syndrome, succeeded to capture 10 diagnostic categories of functional somatic syndromes and somatoform disorders. *J Psychosom Res* 2010; **68**: 415–426. DOI:10.1016/j.jpsychores.2010.02.004

[14] Grundmann O, Yoon SL. Complementary and alternative medicines in irritable bowel syndrome: an integrative view. *World J Gastroenterol* 2014; **20**: 346–362. DOI:10.3748/wjg.v20.i2.346. Review.

[15] Schenström O. Introduction to mindfulness, CD. On the CD he says "It is the most powerful tool that I have come in contact with during my 30 years as a physician" 2006. Available from: http://www.mindfulnesscenter.se

[16] Whorwell PJ, Prior A, Faragher EB. Controlled trial of hypnotherapy in the treatment of severe refractory irritable-bowel syndrome. *Lancet* 1984; **2**: 1232–1234. DOI:10.1016/S0140-6736(84)92793-4

[17] Carolusson S. Dynamic hypnosis, IBS, and the value of individualizing treatment: a clinical perspective. *Int J Clin Exp Hypn* 2014; **62**: 145–163. DOI:10.1080/00207144.2014.869127

[18] Whorwell PJ. Effective management of irritable bowel syndrome – the Manchester Model. *Int J Clin Exp Hypn* 2006; **54**: 21–26. DOI:10.1080/00207140500323006

[19] Whorwell PJ. The history of hypnotherapy and its role in the irritable bowel syndrome. *Aliment Pharmacol Ther* 2005; **22**: 1061–1067. DOI:10.1111/j.1365-2036.2005.02697.x. Review.

[20] Gaylord SA, Palsson OS, Garland EL, Faurot KR, Coble RS, Mann JD, Frey W, Leniek K, Whitehead WE. Mindfulness training reduces the severity of irritable bowel syndrome in women: results of a randomized controlled trial. *Am J Gastroenterol* 2011; **106**:1678–1688. DOI:10.1038/ajg.2011.184

[21] Lahmann C, Röhricht F, Sauer N, Noll-Hussong M, Ronel J, Henrich G, von Arnim A, Loew T. Functional relaxation as complementary therapy in irritable bowel syndrome: a randomized, controlled clinical trial. *J Altern Complement Med* 2010; **16**: 47–52. DOI:10.1089/acm.2009.0084

[22] BAT™, The Institute for Body Awareness Therapy™. Available from: http://www.ibk.nu

[23] Landsman-Dijkstra JJ, van Wijck R, Groothoff JW. The long-term lasting effectiveness on self-efficacy, attribution style, expression of emotions and quality of life of a body

awareness program for chronic a-specific psychosomatic symptoms. *Patient Educ Couns* 2006; **60**: 66–79. PMID:16332472

[24] Eriksson E, Holmquist Å, Wolfgang Bayer W, Bergman B. Blood levels of vitamins, minerals and fatty acids in patients with irritable bowel syndrome (IBS). In proceedings of the European Conference on Psychosomatic Research (ECPR); 27–30 September 2006; Cavtat, Croatia. *J Psychosom Res* 2006; **61**: 422 DOI:10.1016/j.jpsychores.2006.06.004

[25] Welin C, Wilhelmsen L, Welin L, Johansson S, Rosengren A. Perceived health in 50-year-old women and men and the correlation with risk factors, diseases, and symptoms. Gend Med 2011; **8**: 139–149. DOI:10.1016/j.genm.2011.03.005

[26] Eriksson E, Johansson S, Wallander MA, Welin C, Kurlberg G, Eriksson H. Gastrointestinal symptoms in 50 year old women shows a strong correlation to psychosomatics. Continuation of the epidemiological study "Men born 1913". In proceedings of the European Conference on Psychosomatic Research (ECPR); 27–30 September 2006; Cavtat, Croatia. *J Psychosom Res* 2006; **61**: 405–406. DOI:10.1016/j.jpsychores.2006.06.004

[27] Torrestad A, Håkansson M, Axelli T. Development of a program for the treatment of chronic pain and anxiety. A learning process leading from unsound to sound assessment. *Int J Technol Assess Health Care* 1992; **8**: 85–92. PMID:1601597

[28] Moser G. Psychosomatic aspects of bowel diseases. *Z Psychosom Med Psychother* 2006; **52**: 112–126. PMID:16790162

[29] Antonovsky A. The structure and properties of the sense of coherence scale. *Soc Sci Med* 1993; **36**: 725–733. PMID:8480217

[30] Motzer SA, Hertig V, Jarrett M, Heitkemper MM. Sense of coherence and quality of life in women with and without irritable bowel syndrome. *Nurs Res* 2003; **52**: 329–337. PMID:14501547

[31] Sperber AD, Carmel S, Atzmon Y, Weisberg I, Shalit Y, Neumann L, Fich A, Buskila D. The sense of coherence index and the irritable bowel syndrome. A cross-sectional comparison among irritable bowel syndrome patients, with and without coexisting fibromyalgia, irritable bowel syndrome non patients, and controls. *Scand J Gastroenterol* 1999; **34**: 259–263. PMID:10232869

[32] Sephton SE, Sapolsky RM, Kraemer HC, Spiegel D. Diurnal cortisol rhythm as a predictor of breast cancer survival. *J Natl Cancer Inst* 2000; **92**: 994–1000. PMID:10861311

[33] Rosmond R, Bjorntorp P. Low cortisol production in chronic stress. The connection stress-somatic disease is a challenge for future research. *Lakartidningen* 2000; **97**: 4120–4124. PMID:11068377

[34] Gonsalkorale WM, Houghton LA, Whorwell PJ. Hypnotherapy in irritable bowel syndrome: a large-scale audit of a clinical service with examination of factors influencing responsiveness. *Am J Gastroenterol* 2002; **97**: 954–961. PMID:12003432

[35] Gottwald C. Awareness and mindfulness in consciousness-centred body psychotherapy. *Int Body Psychother J* 2014; **13**:67–79. Available from: Academic Search Index, Ipswich, MA.

[36] Lundvik Gyllensten A, Hansson L, Ekdahl C. Patient experiences of basic body awareness therapy and the relationship with the physiotherapist. *J Bodywork Mov Ther* 2003; **7**: 173–183. DOI:10.1111/j.1471-6712.2004.00272.x